DIAGNOSTIC SKILLS
IN
CHINESE MEDICINE

Book 2:

Symptom Analysis and Syndrome Differentiation

By Cat Calhoun, MAcOM, L.Ac.

Cats TCM Notes Press
San Miguel de Allende, Mexico

Diagnostics of Chinese Medicine:
Symptom Analysis and Syndrome Differentiation

For DeLora, my sunshine and my flowers.
Thank you with all my heart for your supporting
and for sticking with me through Chinese Medicine School!

This page intentionally left blank

Diagnostics of Chinese Medicine:
Symptom Analysis and Syndrome Differentiation

Diagnostics of Chinese Medicine:
Symptom Analysis and Syndrome Differentiation

This page intentionally left blank.

Diagnostics of Chinese Medicine:
Symptom Analysis and Syndrome Differentiation

ACKNOWLEDGMENTS

No one does anything truly on their own. I thought myself totally self-sufficient before I dove into the study of Chinese medicine. When that journey began, my eyes opened to the myriads of those who were actively helping me, those who have gone before, and even those who will come long after I'm gone. We are interconnected. You are me, I am you.

I especially want to thank Dr. Song Luo, my teacher and coolest clinical supervisors I had. Such kindness, compassion and wisdom! Thank you for your patience and guidance.

Thank you to Lisa Lapwing, a most awesome practitioner based in Orlando Florida. We studied together, practiced together, we practiced *on* each other in student clinic, and then we became each others' practitioners! Not having Lisa in my daily life is my one giant regret about moving to Mexico.

Thank you to my buds: Donna "Needles" Tatum, Tiffany Chiu Peralez, Vanessa Olsen, Andi Kohn, Mark Hernandez, and Katherine Webster. To Georgie Hoiseth, a kick ass practitioner and fellow computer geek, I thank thee! To Rita Ramirez, I would *NOT* want to be on this journey without you!

To my patients, whom I learn from every day and who trust me with their healthcare, thank you. I love having you in my life.

And to so many more who have loved, supported, and believed in me, I express my gratitude and thanks. May the deity of your choice look favorably upon you all!

Cat Calhoun, MsAcOM, L.Ac

This page intentionally left blank.

Diagnostics of Chinese Medicine:
Symptom Analysis and Syndrome Differentiation

CHAPTER 1
Don't skip this chapter!

You've worked your way through the four diagnostic skills you need to function in clinic. Now we start digging into figuring out how to read patient signs and symptom (s/sx) in order to come up with a working diagnosis and plan of treatment.

This book covers the major diagnostic models you can use to analyze patient s/sx, and how/when to use them. I think it's important to emphasize, especially if you don't have a medical background, that you do not use all of these methods at once. Each of them has their strengths and best usage.

If you're a gamer, you might think of this as getting the codes to the weapons and ammo stash. You can grab as much as you can carry, but you don't use all of your weapons at the same time. You use them strategically.

The same is true for diagnostic methods. These are the methods we are going to cover in this book with the heaviest emphasis on the Zangfu method of diagnosis. Why do we spend so much time on this? Because it's critical for herbal treatment and is probably the hardest to learn. But it's not appropriate for every patient that walks in the door.

Here's a brief overview of what we will cover here.

Diagnostic method	A little bit about that
The Eight Principles	Four pairs of opposites that help you get a bead on what's happening. I use this for complicated cases or for cases that make zero sense when you first look at them. And a little heads up? I still use this several times a week when complex and difficult to sort out sets of s/sx walk in the door! You don't really outgrow this one.
Zangfu Syndromes	We spend a lot of time here, so it seems very heavily emphasized and like maybe you should apply this to every patient. Not necessarily so. It's just complex and has a lot of components to it, so it takes a lot of time.
The Six Stages	Classical method of diagnosis developed by Zhang Zhongjing to categorize, diagnose, and treat febrile diseases that begin with cold invasion.
The Four Levels	Classical method of diagnosis developed by Dr. Ye Tian Shi to categorize, diagnose, and treat febrile diseases that begin with a heat invasion.
The San Jiao	It sounds like a condo complex, but this is another classical method of diagnosing febrile patients that emphasizes the progression of disease through the three jiao: upper, middle, and lower.
Meridian and Collateral theory	Though not covered in this book, meridian and collateral theory is a great way to treat pain. Many practitioners palpate the meridians to find areas of deficiency and excess. You'll cover this in your acupuncture and herbal therapy classes.

SECTION 1
The Eight Principles Diagnostic Model

The Eight Principle Theory is a diagnostic model that uses four pairs of inseparable, interconnected, and complimentary opposites to help you get a handle on what is happening with your patient.

Though it seems deceptively simple, this method is a great way to start when you are presented with a patient with really confusing symptoms. Honestly, I still use it all the time, even after all this time.

Why else should you learn this diagnostic method? It's heavily tested on the US national boards and therefore in most Chinese medicine curriculums taught in the US.

Pay specific attention to anything **bolded in this book,** as bolded stuff is very likely to show up on quizzes and national boards. Other stuff will too, but this is almost guaranteed.

This page intentionally left blank.

Diagnostics of Chinese Medicine:
Symptom Analysis and Syndrome Differentiation

CHAPTER 2
Exterior and Interior

The Exterior and Interior pair describes the location (depth) and stage of the disease (early, mid, or late) as well as the direction it is traveling (interior to exterior or exterior to interior). You do this by using your skills to observe the signs and symptoms you see and feel, so pay particular attention to knowing these, especially to what you see **in bold type**!

> **The Exterior and Interior pair describes the location and stage of the disease as well as the direction it is traveling.**

As an example, a disease might be on the exterior and migrating inward. This also tells you the stage of a disease. Using this same example, you now know that this is not the beginning stage, but the early middle stage.

EXTERIOR SYNDROMES

Exterior syndromes are located in the superficial (Yang) portions of the body. Specifically, the superficial part of the body is the skin, hair, muscles and interspaces between the muscles, and in the meridians and collateral channels.

An exterior syndrome also describes the *early* stage of a disease. They are generally characterized as coming on suddenly and being short in duration.

An exterior syndrome refers to a **group of pathological conditions resulting from invasion of superficial portion of body by exogenous pathogenic factors**.

- Exogenous refers to pathogenic factors originating from outside the body

- "Syndrome" refers to a grouping of symptoms.

This table details what you need to know about exterior syndromes.

Things to know about exterior syndromes	Specifics
Cause	Invasion of exogenous pathogenic factors
Location	Superficial portion of the body
Nature	• **Sudden onset of symptoms** • **Short duration** • **Early stage of an exogenous disease**
Chief Manifestations (general s/sx)	• **Intolerance (aversion) to cold, wind, and chill.** • **Fever simultaneous with chills** • Tongue: thin coating • Pulse: superficial
Accompanying s/sx	• Headache • General body aches • Nasal obstruction and/or discharge • Sneezing • Coughing

Types of Exterior Syndromes

One can get any of the four types of exterior syndromes. They are:

- Exterior heat syndrome
- Exterior cold syndrome
- Exterior excess syndrome
- Exterior deficiency syndrome

We have talked about at length about heat and cold signs and symptoms in *Chinese Medicine 101,*[1] *Chinese Medicine 102,*[2] and in the first diagnostics book, *Diagnostic Skills in Chinese Medicine – Book 1: The Four Diagnostic Skills.*[3] You probably know what heat and cold look like by now. Add the exterior signs and symptoms to that and you have a pretty good picture of what exterior heat and cold syndromes look like.

We'll talk about the excess and deficiency syndrome specifics in just a minute.

Treating an Exterior Syndrome

The basic treatment principle is to expel the exterior pathogen/s. Sometimes this is called "dispersing," keeping the pathogen/s from ganging up and kicking ass.

Acupuncture opens the meridians and expels the pathogens. Points on the head, arm, and upper back - the yang areas – do this rather effectively. You can also do cupping on the shoulders and upper back to help draw the pathogens back to the surface and disperse them.

Herbal therapy generally consists of leaves and twigs. Light herbs will easily disperse disease from the superficial areas. Herbs such as jin yin hua (honeysuckle flowers), bo he (peppermint), fang feng (root of the siler plant), and xin yi hua (the fuzzy part from the inside of the magnolia flower) are several of the go-to herbs for exterior syndromes.

---

[1] *Chinese Medicine 101: Start with the Foundations* (ISBN: 1093826703), available on Amazon.com in both digital and paperback format.

[2] *Chinese Medicine 102: Complete Your Foundations* (ISBN: 1095324306), available on Amazon.com in both digital and paperback format.

[3] *Diagnostic Skills in Chinese Medicine – Book 1: The Four Diagnostic Skills* (ISBN: 1096340577), available on Amazon.com in both digital and paperback format.

Fang feng is kind of unusual – roots don't generally expel the exterior. This one is used with jing jie (Japanese catnip) to expel wind from the superficial parts of the body, which will take other pathogens along for the ride and leave the body.

INTERIOR SYNDROMES

The location of an interior syndrome is in the five Zang and six Fu organs, the Yin areas of the body. To say a patient has an interior syndrome is to define the *stage* of the disease. It also indicates the *direction* a disease is traveling. For instance, if a disease starts as an exterior syndrome and then progresses to an interior syndrome, you have defined the direction the disease is traveling in the body.

An interior syndrome refers to:

1. **Pathological conditions resulting from transmission of exogenous pathogenic factors to the interior of body, which affects functions of Zangfu organs**.

2. **Functional disturbances of Zangfu** organs resulting in an interior set of signs and symptoms (a syndrome) rather than from a disease progression from exterior to interior.

This table details what you need to know about interior syndromes.

Things to know about interior syndromes	Specifics
Causes	• **Transmission** of a persistent pathogen from exterior to interior Zangfu organs • **Direct attack** on the Zangfu by exogenous pathogens • Lifestyle factors affecting the Zangfu organs directly leading to functional

	disturbances of the organ/s (ie., drastic emotional changes, improper diet, stress, overwork, etc.)
Location	Interior, Zangfu (organ level) of the body.
Nature	• Chronic in nature - of longer duration than an acute disease • Could describe the mid or late stage of a disease
Chief Manifestations	• Mainly appear in/on the trunk or Zangfu organs. (Constipation, stomach ache, palpitations, diarrhea, etc.) • Tongue: yellow or black coating with a slippery or greasy texture, body could be purplish, pale, trembling, deviated and more, depending on the organ/s affected. • Pulses: vary depending on manifestation, but could see deep, slippery, wiry, choppy, and more.

Clinically, interior syndromes could be interior cold, interior heat, interior deficiency, or interior excess. We have and will talk about cold and heat quite a lot. Deficiency and excess are the next big topic on the hit parade.

Treatment options are all over the map for interior syndromes and they will depend on the organ/s affected. It's common to use points on the chest, back, leg, and foot as well as combinations of the back shu and front mu points as well as the lower he-sea points and source points. More on all of those in energetics and point location studies. Herbal therapies generally rely on seeds, heavy herbs, and roots, which are more associated with yin and interior.

DIFFERENTIATION OF EXTERIOR AND INTERIOR SYNDROMES

Here is how to tell them apart. The big thing to know here is the fever s/sx. In the interior syndrome, the fever is definitely an either or. If there is fever, there is no aversion to cold. If there *is* aversion to cold, there's no fever.

Exterior syndrome	Interior syndrome
Fever + aversion to cold	**Fever + no aversion to cold** *--or--* **Aversion to cold + *no* fever**
Thin white tongue coating	Abnormal qualities of coatings
Superficial pulse	Deep pulse

Know this fever thang!

RELATIONSHIP BETWEEN EXTERIOR AND INTERIOR SYNDROMES

Exterior syndromes always want to go deeper into the body, getting past the defenses and breaking into the supply lines so they can party at our expense. Fortunately, the body can also uses the same routes to push the pathogens out.

Here are two things to know about this relationship between this pair of complementary opposites:

1. **Pathogens are transmitted from exterior to interior.**
   Example: An illness starts with slight aversion to cold and a fever. Progresses to no aversion to cold, but aversion to heat with thirst, dark urine, thick yellow tongue coat, deeper pulse. This is a progression from external to internal.

   Prognosis becomes worse as the disease goes from out to in. Why would a pathogen migrate inward?
   a. Weakened body resistance to diseases
       Starting with a deficiency, basically.

   b. Hyperactivity of pathogens
       Very strong pathogens, virulent disease.

c. Improper care, incorrect or delayed treatment
    If you don't diagnose the problem correctly and treat
    it from a poor diagnosis, you can make the problem
    far worse. As an example, if you miss the heat signs
    and diagnose an exterior heat invasion as an exterior
    cold invasion, you will likely introduce more heat
    into the body with herbs and treatment methods and
    make the problem worse.

    Well meaning but poorly trained people do this all
    the time. That's why acupuncture lobbying groups
    are so vocal about chiropractors, physical therapists,
    and MDs who receive extremely cursory training (if
    they get training at all) practicing dry needling,
    which is just a marketing term for acupuncture.

2. **Pathogens are transmitted from interior to exterior.
   Prognosis is good**, as this indicates improvement. The
   pulse is not so deep and the tongue coat gets thinner.
   Why would this happen?
   a. Correct treatment
   b. Good care
   c. Strengthened resistance to disease.

This page intentionally left blank.
I meant to do that.....yeah, that's it.

Diagnostics of Chinese Medicine:
          Symptom Analysis and Syndrome Differentiation

CHAPTER 3
Heat and Cold

These terms describe the nature and stage of a disease. The *Neijing* says that a predominance of Yang gives rise to heat as it accumulates; a predominance of Yin gives rise to cold as it accumulates.

HEAT SYNDROMES

Heat Syndromes are **pathological conditions caused by invasion of exogenous pathogenic heat or by Yin deficiency** in the interior (leading to deficient heat).

Heat syndromes belong to Yang. If they are caused by an exogenous heat pathogen, they are acute and urgent. If they are caused by deficiency of Yin, they are chronic and long-term.

Heat syndromes, like Exterior and Interior syndromes, can arise from an external pathogen or from a functional interior problem that arises either from a pathogen traveling from outer to inner or from bad lifestyle choices.

General s/sx of a heat syndrome

There are some symptoms commonly associated with heat syndromes. These are true for both deficient and full heat, though with deficient heat the symptoms will be less due to the depleted condition – less tongue coat, red face but only at the cheekbones, etc.

- **Fever**
- **Thirst, wants cold drink**
- Iritability
- **Constipation**
- **Red tongue body, yellow dry coating**
- Preference for coolness
- **Red face and eyes**
- **Restlesness**
- **Dark yellow, scanty urine**
- **Rapid pulse**

Clinically, you could see exterior heat syndromes, interior heat syndromes, excess heat syndrome, and deficient heat syndromes. Treatment of heat syndromes varies depending on these types. Notice the "expel heat" in the case of exterior and excess heat versus the "clear heat" terminology of the interior and deficient forms of heat. This is not an accident! You will see these terms associated in this way often.

Heat Syndrome	Treatment
Exterior heat	Expel heat pathogen
Interior heat	Clear heat
Excess heat	Expel heat pathogen
Deficient heat	Tonify Yin + clear heat

COLD SYNDROMES

Cold Syndromes are pathological conditions resulting from exposure to exogenous pathogenic cold or from deficiency of yang (or yin excess) in the interior of body.

Cold syndromes are Yin in nature and could affect the interior and/or the exterior. Durations of cold syndromes could be long or short, depending on the manifestation. If the cold syndrome is affecting the exterior of the body, the duration of the disease will be short. If this is affecting the interior, it's a longer-term, chronic condition.

General s/sx of a cold syndrome

- **Aversion to cold**
- No thirst
- **Pallor**/pale face
- **Loose stool**
- **Pale tongue body, white moist coating**

- Preference for warmth
- Bland taste in the mouth
- **Cold limbs**
- **Clear urine, more profuse**
- **Slow or tense pulse**

Clinically, you could see the following expressions of a cold syndrome:

Cold Syndrome	Treatment
Exterior cold	Expel cold
Interior cold	Warm it
Excess cold	Expel cold
Deficient cold	Warm it

COMPARISON BETWEEN HEAT AND COLD SYNDROMES

Let's do a comparison chart of cold vs. heat to help you see the differences.

	Cold s/sx	Heat s/sx
Aversions	Aversion to cold, prefers heat	Aversion to heat, prefers cool
Thirst	No	Yes, wants cold
Face	Pale	Red
Limbs	Cold	Warm
Stools	Loose	Dry, constipated
Urine	Profuse/clear	Scanty, dark, reddish
Tongue	Pale, greasy white fur*	Red, yellow fur*
Pulse	Slow, tight	Fast

*FUR?! Yes, fur. This is another fun TCM terminology thing. Fur is the same thing as coating. And no, I'm not messing with you.

RELATIONSHIP BETWEEN COLD AND HEAT SYNDROMES

Two interrelationships to know between these two types of syndromes:

1. **Cold transforms to heat.**
   Cold syndrome occurs first and gradually changes into heat. Example: Patient starts with an aversion to cold, general body aching and no sweating. Then aversion to cold subsides, fever persists, the patient becomes irritable, thirst increases, the tongue body gets red and the coating ("fur") gets yellow, etc.

2. **Heat transforms to cold.**
   Heat s/sx come first then gradually changes to cold.
   Example: Patient with a heat syndrome of some variety
   suddenly starts having cold limbs, complexion takes on
   a pallor, and the pulse becomes deep and slow.

COMBINATION SYNDROMES S/SX

OK, we've talked exterior/interior and heat/cold, so let's talk
combinations of these syndromes so far.

Pay attention to these charts! Spend some time writing them out
and comparing the s/sx. I've created all the charts below with
the same s/sx categories so you can do this when you study. If
you see no answer in the charts, that means there's no specific
s/sx that goes with that.

Exterior + Heat Syndromes

Exterior + heat is also referred to in Chinese medicine as "wind
heat." This is an exogenous heat attacking the superficial
portions of the body.

Exterior + Heat	S/sx
Fever/chills	Fever
Aversions	Slight intolerance to wind/cold
Pain sensations	Headache
Thirst	Slight thirst for cold, dry sensation in mouth
Sweating	Possibly
Complexion	Face could be reddish
Energy level	
Limbs	Warm
Urine	
Stool	
Tongue	Red tip and edges
Pulse	Superficial, rapid

Exterior + Cold Syndromes

Exterior + cold in Chinese medicine is also referred to as "wind cold." (Wind is often the "carrier" – we all have that one friend in the group who talks us into lord knows what and we go along with it. Wind is that friend!

Exterior + Cold	S/sx
Fever/chills	Fever, but chills are more
Aversions	Massive intolerance to cold
Pain sensations	General aching
Thirst	No!
Sweating	*No!*
Complexion	
Energy level	
Limbs	
Urine	
Stool	
Tongue	Thin, white, moist tongue coating
Pulse	Superficial, tight

Side by side comparison of these two:

Category	Exterior heat	Exterior cold
Fever/chills	Fever	Fever, but chills are more
Aversions	Slight intolerance to wind/cold	Huge intolerance to cold
Pain	Headache	General aching
Thirst	Slight thirst for cold, dry sensation in mouth	No
Sweating	Possibly	No
Complexion	Face could be reddish	
Energy		
Limbs	Warm	
Stool		
Tongue		Thin, white, moist tongue coating
Pulse	Red tip and edges	Superficial, tight
	Superficial, rapid	

Interior + Heat Syndrome

Interior heat is generally caused by an exterior pathogen that is transmitted to the interior and changes to heat *or* heat pathogens that attack the interior organs directly.

Interior syndromes, whether of the heat or cold varieties, *can be either excess or deficient in nature.* We'll get more specific about excess and deficiency in the next chapter. Compare the s/sx below to each other so you can see the difference.

Category	Excess interior heat s/sx	Xu interior heat s/sx*
Fever/chills	High fever	Palm/sole heat*
Aversions		
Pain	Possible abdominal distention, worse with pressure	
Thirst	Strong thirst, wants cold beverages	Thirst, dry throat*
Sweating		Night sweating*
Complexion	Red face, red eyes	Red in zygomatic area (also called malar flush)*
Psycho/emo	Irritable, poss delirium	
Energy level		
Limbs		
Urine	Scanty, red	
Stool	Constipation, dry	
Other		
Tongue	Red body, yellow dry coat	Thin red body, less/ mapped/mirror coating*
Pulse	Flood, slippery, fast	Thin, fast*

*Know these! These are Yin deficient heat signs.
You will see these over and over and over ......

Diagnostics of Chinese Medicine:
Symptom Analysis and Syndrome Differentiation

Interior + Cold Syndromes

Interior cold is caused by cold pathogens attacking the Zangfu directly *or* it is a deficiency of Yang Qi.

You see the Yang xu signs in the Xu interior cold column below.

Again, interior syndromes can be either deficient or excess in nature. Compare the s/sx below to each other so you can see the difference. I've provided the same s/sx categories as you found in the interior heat syndromes chart so you can lay them out and compare then when you study.

Category	Excess interior cold s/sx (Yin excess)	Xu interior cold s/sx (Yang deficiency)
Fever/chills		
Aversions		
Pain	Abdominal cold pain, worse with pressure	Abdominal cold pain, better with pressure
Thirst		No, but does prefer warm beverages.
Sweating		
Complexion	Pale/pallor	Pale
Psycho/emo		
Energy level		Fatigued, sluggish
Limbs	Cold, prefers warmth	Cold
Urine	Clear	Profuse, clear
Stool	Loose	Loose
Other	Bland taste, profuse saliva	Shortness of breath (noted as SOB in charts)
Tongue	Pale, white coating	Pale, moist white coat
Pulse	Deep, slow, tight	Deep, weak, slow

True Heat with False Cold &
True Cold with False Heat

Just when you're getting the hang of this, I'm going to toss a bomb into your well-organized thoughts.

Under normal circumstances, the warm and cool elements in your body mix, giving you a pleasant overall feeling in your internal temperature world. But if there is too much heat in the body, the cold gets pushed to the outer edges of the body, the head and the limbs. The same thing happens with cold – if there is too much, then the heat gets pushed to the outer edges of the body.

Something similar happens in the environment. Summer storms are a great example of this. The weather is hot in Texas in the late summer/early fall already, but right before a summer storm blows in (often bringing tornados and hail), it gets even hotter and more miserable than normal. I mean, it's horrid. Then you see the edge of the storm front and the temperatures begin to drop rapidly, sometimes by as much as 40 degrees. I've had on shorts one minute and a parka the next on more than one occasion!

Why does this happen? There are two competing air masses – one hot and one cold. When the temperature difference between the two is a big difference like this, there's no way they can mix easily. One air mass is simply going to push the other around until osmosis can do its' job and even things out.

The same thing happens in the body. The rush of internal heat or cold can't mix quickly enough with the native internal environment, so the opposing temperature gets pushed to the edges. That's when interior cold starts looking a lot like heat. . . and interior heat starts looking a lot like cold. . . . until you look deeper.

Always look at the s/sx that affect the *interior* of the body. These will tell you the truth. Notice the difference between the feeling of the body and the limbs. This is something *you feel* using your new, awesome palpation skills, covered in Book 1.[4] The condition of the body tells you the real internal temperature excess. You also see it in the throat, thirst, urine, stool, tongue, and pulse. The limbs and the complexion are lying to you, even if they don't mean to! ☺

Category	Interior (true) heat + False cold signs	Interior cold (true) + False heat signs
Body feels...	Hot	Cold
Limbs feel...	Cold	Warm or hot
Throat feels...	Dry	Not dry
Thirst	Yes, wants cold drink	Yes, wants warm drink
Complexion	Pale	Red
Urine	Scanty, dark, reddish	Profuse, clear color
Stool	Dry	Loose
Other	Doesn't want to be covered up	Wants to be covered up
Tongue	Deep red, yellow coat	Pale, white moist coat
Pulse	Deep, forceful	Large, weak

Know how to tell the difference between true heat/false cold and true cold/false heat!

---

[4] Chapter 13, *Diagnostic Skills in Chinese Medicine – Book 1: The Four Diagnostic Skills* (ISBN: 1096340577), available on Amazon.com in both digital and paperback format.

This page intentionally left blank.
You're welcome.
I don't know what for.

CHAPTER 4
Excess and Deficiency

Deficiency or Excess expresses the relative *strength* of the pathogens and of the anti-pathogenic Qi. The short version of this whole section: Excess refers to the strength of the pathogen. Deficiency here refers to lack of strength of the Zheng or Correct/Upright Qi of the patient. Now let's explore this in more detail.

EXCESS SYNDROME

As a general rule, excess refers to the strength or hyperactivity of the evil or the disease. I mean, seriously, if the Zheng Qi was in excess, this patient would be well, right?

Syndromes of excess refer to pathological conditions in which the pathogenic factor is hyperactive, *and* the antipathogenic qi remains strong. The reasons for an excess syndrome? 1) An attacking external evil and 2) a dysfunction of the internal organs in some way.

General symptoms of excess syndromes:
- Agitation
- Pain that is aggravated by pressure
- Constipation or tenesmus
- Dysuria
- Loud, sonorous voice
- Distention and fullness of chest/abdomen
- Coarse breathing
- Thick, sticky tongue coating
- Excess type pulse[5]

Treatment is to expel the pathogens with acupuncture, cupping, herbs, and reducing methods.

---

[5] Section 4, *Diagnostic Skills in Chinese Medicine – Book 1: The Four Diagnostic Skills* (ISBN: 1096340577), available on Amazon.com in both digital and paperback format.

Patients might have several combinations of heat/cold, exterior/interior, and excess/deficiency. If you want the s/sx, refer back to Chapter 2 and 3 for information in hot/cold, exterior/interior. The signs and symptoms are all listed there.

It's actually a bit redundant to say "exterior excess heat" because this is the same thing as an exterior heat. And it's the same thing as wind heat invasion. In the same way, excess exterior cold = exterior cold = wind cold invasion.

DEFICIENCY SYNDROME

"Deficiency" here refers to the lack of strength of the Zheng Qi, aka, the Correct Qi or the antipathogenic Qi. The *Neijing* says, "When Correct Qi exists, evil cannot attack you." In another place it states, "The reason evil Qi attacks is patient's Qi must be deficient."

Yin, Yang, Qi, and Blood can all be affected by deficiency. General symptoms of a deficiency look like the ones in the table below. Something that is true for any of the syndromes we've talked about (or ever will talk about) is that you won't see *all* of these signs and symptoms in one patient. I've indicated the general symptoms and then pointed out what that s/sx would be a deficiency *of*.

Know the general s/sx!!

S/sx	What kind of xu that might indicate
Emaciation	Yin xu, often
Listlessness – lacking zeal or enthusiasm	General xu s/sx
Lassitude – weakness, exhaustion, wearinss	General xu s/sx
Feeble breathing	Lung Qi xu
Dislike of speaking	Lung Qi xu
Pallor	Qi xu, Blood xu, Yang xu
Palpitations	Heart Qi xu, Zong Qi xu
Shortness of breath (SOB)	Lung Qi xu, Zong Qi xu
Insomnia	Heart Qi xu and/or Heart Blood xu

Poor memory	Heart Blood xu
Spontaneous sweating*	Qi and/or Yang xu
Night sweats	Qi xu and/or Yin xu
Nocturnal emissions	Yin xu, Qi xu, Yang xu
Nocturnal enuresis (involuntary passing of urine)	Kidney Qi xu (most common reason for bedwetting)
Pain is alleviated by pressure	General xu s/sx
Dry tongue	Indicates xu has led to body fluid damage
No to little tongue coating	Yin xu
Deficiency type pulses[6]	Section 4 of previous book
Tremors	Liver xu Note: tremors can also be caused by excesses such as external wind invasions or internal excesses such as rising Liver Yang or rising Liver Fire.

*See that "spontaneous sweating" symptom? That's pretty definitive for a deficiency. The body is designed to be able to control the sweating pores – the defensive Qi is responsible for this. When the Correct/defensive Qi is weak however, it cannot control the sweating pores, so they kind of "leak" spontaneously. This is a wimpy sweat that won't help push out pathogens, so it does the body no good.

Note that in the excess syndrome discussion, you saw zero sweating! That's because the Correct Qi is healthy and can open and shut those "doors" as needed. Unfortunately, pathogens take advantage of this. If they successfully invade, they slam those pores shut so they can stay inside. Therefore, no sweating. When this is true you *can* use herbs to induce sweating and push the pathogen out, but that's hella inappropriate in the case of a deficiency syndrome as it will just weaken the body further.

Yang deficiency and Yin deficiency specific s/sx

Yang, Yin, Qi, and Blood deficiency all have more specific presentations (s/sx) you also need to know. In addition to the possible list of general syndromes, you will add these.

---

[6] Section 4, *Diagnostic Skills in Chinese Medicine – Book 1: The Four Diagnostic Skills* (ISBN: 1096340577), available on Amazon.com in both digital and paperback format.

It seems wise to put these in a comparison chart so you can see the difference between the two. We've talked in both foundations and diagnostics about yin and yang deficiency s/sx, so hopefully this is starting to feel familiar.

Category	Yang deficiency (with xu cold)	Yin deficiency (with xu heat)
Temperature	Chills	Heat in palms/soles
Limbs	Cold	Warm/normal
Body	Could be puffy or normal	**Emaciation**
Complexion	Pale	Malar flush
Energy level	Listlessness/lassitude	(not necessarily affected)
Fevers	(none)	Tidal/afternoon fever
Sweating	Spontaneous sweats	Spontaneous and night sweats
Thirst	None	Dry throat and mouth
Urine	Profuse and clear	Darker yellow
Stools	Diarrhea about 5am	Dry
Tongue	Pale body, white coat	**Red body, little coat**
Pulse	Deep, weak, slow	**Thready, rapid**

Qi deficiency and Blood deficiency specific s/sx

Category	Qi deficiency	Blood deficiency
Vision	*(unaffected)*	Blurred
Complexion	*(varies)*	Pale – complexion, eyelids, gums, nails, lips, mouth all pale
Memory/ concentration	*(unaffected)*	Poor memory, poor concentration
Energy level	Fatigue, Lassitude	Fatigue
Menstruation	*(varies)*	Irregular, scanty
Sweating	Spontaneous	*(unaffected)*
Other	Shortness of breath Weak voice	Dizziness
Tongue	Swollen body, teethmarks, white coat	**Pale body, white coat**
Pulse	Weak, soft	**Weak, soft**

Diagnostics of Chinese Medicine:
Symptom Analysis and Syndrome Differentiation

1. You can have a combination of deficiency and excess. This is when the antipathogenic Qi is deficient and the pathogen is excessive at the same time.

2. Excess can lead to deficiency
   The excess condition can deplete the resources.
   As an example, a patient that starts with The Four Bigs (fever, thirst, sweating and pulse) over time moves into emaciation, poor energy and feebleness, the tongue coating gets very thin, and they develop a thread, weak pulse.

3. Deficiency can become an excess.
   For instance, you have a patient with a Sp Qi xu with s/sx of fullness after eating, generalized fatigue, loose stools, shortness of breath, a swollen tongue with a white coat, and a weak pulse.

   This patient will then be susceptible to pathogens, such as damp retention, which would be an excess. This person might develop clear phlegm and a cough, edema in the legs, a tongue with teethmarks and a thick greasy coat, and a slippery pulse.

This page intentionally left blank

Diagnostics of Chinese Medicine:
Symptom Analysis and Syndrome Differentiation

CHAPTER 5
Yang and Yin

Yin and Yang are the primary and underlying principle of this method of diagnosing. All of the pairs are some expression of Yin and Yang.

And I know most of the time we *say* Yin and Yang, but you will note below that each pair is listed with the Yang expression first and the Yin expression second. This is because Yang is the active principle and is the first to manifest in disease and disharmony states.

All of the pairs in the preceding chapters dedicated to the Eight Principles are Yang/Yin associated! An exterior excess heat, for instance is truly a Yang exterior excess heat. A interior cold deficiency is an Yang interior cold deficiency. See what I mean?

The big danger is that Yin and Yang will be impacted to the point that they collapse due to imbalances. When either Yin or Yang is sufficiently damaged, the Yin Yang pair bond is broken and the body can die. These are referred to as Yang and Yin collapses. Here are the s/sx of each collapse. **Know them!**

Category	Yang Collapse s/sx	Yin Collapse s/sx
Sweating	Profuse, cold, no taste	Sticky, hot, salty
Hot/cold	Cold body and limbs	Fever in body, warm limbs
Breathing	Weak	Shortness of breath
Spirit	Listless	Irritability, restlessness
Thirst, drinking	No thirst, when drinks wants warm	Yes, when drinks wants cold
Tongue	Pale, moist	Red, dry
Pulse	Very weak	Rapid, weak

Here's a little symptom wrap-up for you with the Yang and Yin parts thrown in. Nothing new to learn, just a comparison chart.

	Nature	Main s/sx	Tongue	Pulse
Yang	Exterior	Aversion to cold Fever Aching in head/body	Thin white or yellow coat	Floating/ Superficial
	Heat	Fever Thirst for cold drinks Flushed face Red eyes Scanty yellow urine Constipation	Red tongue body, dry yellow coating	Rapid
	Excess	Hyperactive Hoarse breathing Pain/fullness in ab/chest More pain with touch Difficult urination Dry stool	Thick, greasy coating	Forceful
Yin	Interior	Same as interior excess and xu	Thick	Deep
	Cold	Aversion to cold Likes warmth Pale face Cold limbs Clear urine Loose stools	Pale body, moist white coating	Slow
	Xu	Pale face Lassitude Dull pain Palpitations Weakness Spontaneous sweating Touch/press feels good Shortness of breath Thin body	Very little to no coating	Thin

Diagnostics of Chinese Medicine:
Symptom Analysis and Syndrome Differentiation

So how do you use all of this information? You look at the pairs – exterior/interior, excess/deficiency, heat/cold – and you add up the information you get. Signs and symptoms of an exterior invasion, deficiency in the body, and heat lead you to the conclusion that a body with deficient defensive Qi is trying to fight off an exterior heat invasion. S/sx of an interior deficient cold would guide you into another arena of treatment.

That might be sufficient to give you a treatment strategy and you're off to the races. Or it might guide you to an internal syndrome that needs a little more exploration. You might decide there's a yin deficiency of some kind with deficient heat signs. What organ or organs are affected? This won't really tell you, so you would need to jump to a Zangfu type diagnosis model. You could discover that this started with an exterior cold a week ago and is now showing heat signs, so you jump to the Six Channels method to figure out where it's going and what stage the disease is in, which will inform your treatment methods a little differently.

See what I mean? This can point you in the right direction and (once you have a little experience in your pocket) it's a fast way to evaluate the basics, especially in the face of a bunch of weird symptoms and signs that don't seem to make sense.

Honestly, that's when I use it the most! I've had a number patients who come in with a long list of symptoms which they will rapid fire at me because they've been to a dozen practitioners of varying flavors for the same issues, so this list is on the tip of their tongues from having repeated it so often. Many times, diagnoses from other practitioners are tossed in to this list. This can get overwhelming and confusing if you let it. No big. Write it out Eight Principles style and move on.

This also tells you if you are seeing a Yang based disease or a Yin based disease, which again, is the dominant principle in this method of diagnosis.

Study Guide for Section 1

Eight Principles Study Questions

Question	Answer
What does "differentiation of syndromes" mean in TCM?	Method of recognizing and diagnosing diseases.
What is the Eight Principle Theory?	Eight basic categories (in pairs) of syndromes used to analyze pathologies for differentiation.
Name the 4 pairs of eight in the Eight Principle Theory.	1. Yin-Yang 2. Interior-Exterior 3. Cold-Heat 4. Deficient-Excess
What does Yin-Yang represent in the Eight Principle Theory?	Yin-Yang is the chief principle.
What does Interior-Exterior show in the Eight Principle Theory?	This is the location and stage of the disease.
What information does Cold-Heat give you?	The nature and stage of the disease.
What information does Deficiency-Excess provide in the Eight Principle Theory?	The relative strength of the pathogens and antipathogenic Qi.
Give the possible Exterior locations in the Eight Principle Theory.	1. Skin 2. Hair 3. Muscles and interspaces 4. Superficial portions of meridians/collaterals
What locations of a disease would be considered Interior per the Eight Principle Theory?	Five zang and six fu.

How does the Eight Principle Theory help you determine the depth and development of a disease's development?	By determining previous and current locations of a disease (Exterior or Interior) you can determine where the disease is at the moment and what direction it is traveling—going internal or getting better and becoming more external.
Define Exterior syndrome.	Group of pathological conditions and symptoms resulting from the invasion of the superficial portion of the body by exogenous pathogens.
What is the cause of an exterior syndrome?	Invasion of exogenous pathogenic factors
What is the general location of an Exterior Syndrome?	Superficial portion of the body (skin, hair, muscles and interspaces, superficial portions of the channels/collaterals)
What is the onset and duration of an exterior syndrome? What stage of exogenous disease does this represent?	Onset: sudden Duration: short Stage: early stage
What are the chief manifestations of Exterior Syndromes?	1. Intolerance to cold, wind and chill 2. Fever to go along with the chills 3. Thin tongue coating 4. Superficial/floating pulse
What other symptoms might you see that would lead you to conclude that this is an Exterior Syndrome?	• Headache • General aching • Nasal obstruction and discharge • Sneezing • Cough

What 4 "flavors" of Exterior Syndromes might you see?	• Exterior cold • Exterior heat • Exterior excess • Exterior deficiency
What treatment principles could you employ for Exterior Syndromes?	Expel the pathogen, disperse it to keep the evil from coming further in to the body.
What is an Interior Syndrome?	Pathological condition resulting from transmission of exogenous pathogens to interior where it affects the zangfu. Can also be a result of the functional disturbances of the zangfu.
Give 3 causes of an Internal Syndrome.	1. Transmission of persistent pathogens from exterior to interior to invade zangfu. 2. Direct attack on Zangfu by external pathogen (skipping the Exterior step) 3. Drastic emotional changes, improper diet, overstrain, stress which lead to functional disturbances of the zangfu.
What is the location of an internal syndrome?	Zangfu organs
Is an interior syndrome generally acute or chronic?	Chronic
What kind of duration would you expect to see in an Internal Syndrome?	Long, chronic type
What stages of a disease does an Interior Syndrome represent?	Middle or late stage
Where do symptoms appear in an Interior Syndrome?	On the trunk of the body in the location of the zangfu organ(s) affected.

What kind of pulses do you see in Interior Syndromes?	Deep, slippery, wiry, choppy
What are the 4 kinds of Interior Syndromes?	1. Interior cold 2. Interior heat 3. Interior excess 4. Interior deficiency
What are the 3 things you can use to determine if a disease is Exterior or Interior?	1. Fever and aversion to cold 2. Tongue coatings 3. Pulse quality

What are the differences in fever and aversion to cold status you see between the Exterior and Interior syndromes?	• Exterior:
	Fever + aversion to cold
	• Interior:
	  o Fever with *no aversion to cold*…..OR
	  o Aversion to cold with *no fever*

Which syndrome displays a thin white tongue coating: Interior or Exterior?	• Exterior
What is the difference in pulse quality between Interior and Exterior syndromes?	• Exterior = superficial • Interior = deep
Describe the progression of symptoms when an Exterior syndrome becomes and Interior syndrome.	Exterior symptoms include fever with slight aversion to cold. When pathogen moves to interior, changes to aversion to heat with thirst, dark urine. Tongue coating will change. Pulse will go from superficial to deep.
Four reasons a pathogen would progress from exterior to interior.	• Weakened body resistance to disease • Hyperactivity/strength of pathogens • Improper care • Incorrect or delayed treatment

What is the prognosis when a pathogen goes from exterior to interior?	Not so great
What happens to the tongue coat and pulse when a disease goes from Interior to Exterior? What is the prognosis?	• Tongue coat: from thick to thin • Pulse: gets less deep • Prognosis: good!
3 reasons a disease would migrate from inward to outward?	• Correct treatment • Good care • Strengthened resistance to disease
What 2 principles in the Eight Principle Theory would be used to differentiate the nature and stage of a disease?	Cold-Heat
Per the Neijing, what gives predominance to heat and what gives predominance to cold?	Heat: Yang Cold: Yin
What are cold syndromes and what do they result from?	Pathological conditions resulting from: • Exogenous pathogenic cold • Deficiency of yang in the interior.
What 2 areas can be affected by Cold Syndromes and what are the expected durations in each of those areas?	Exterior - short duration Interior – longer duration
What 4 types (clinical manifestations) can you see in Cold Syndromes	• Exterior cold • Interior cold • Excess cold (too much Yin) • Deficiency cold (lack of Yang)
What is the definition of a Heat Syndrome?	• invasion of exogenous pathogenic heat....OR... • deficiency of Yin in the body's interior

By nature, is a Heat Syndrome yin or yang?	Yang
If a Heat Syndrome is caused by exogenous heat, what is the nature of that condition?	Acute and urgent in nature
If a Heat Syndrome is caused by a deficiency of some kind, what is the nature of the syndrome?	Chronic
Is a Heat Syndrome internal or external in nature?	Can be either
So, in summary, what are the 4 natures of a Heat Syndrome?	• Belongs to Yang • Acute and urgent in nature if caused by exogenous heat. • Chronic in nature if caused by a deficiency of yin, yang, qi, blood. • Can be either an external (short duration) or internal (long duration) syndrome.
What differences in symptoms will you notice if the heat in the heat syndrome is a deficient heat?	Less of everything—lower fever, less thirst, redness in the face will be limited to zygomatic region, tongue coat will be thinner, etc.
What 4 clinical manifestations can you see with heat syndromes? What are the recommended treatments?	1. Exterior heat 2. Interior heat 3. Excess heat 4. Deficient heat
What are the two relationships between Cold and Heat Syndromes?	• A Cold Syndrome will eventually become a Heat Syndrome. • A Heat Syndrome will eventually become a Cold Syndrome.

Why might a Heat Syndrome become a Cold syndrome?	Either a constitutional Yang deficiency and/or an exhaustion of Yang Qi during the course of the illness.
What are the 4 combination Exterior-Interior/Cold-Heat Syndromes?	1. Exterior cold 2. Exterior heat 3. Interior cold 4. Interior heat
Please define an Exterior Cold syndrome	A group of syndromes caused by exogenous cold attacking the superficial portion of the body.
Please define Exterior Heat Syndrome?	A group of syndromes caused by exogenous heat attacking the superficial portion of the body.
Define interior cold syndrome	Group of syndromes caused by: • cold pathogens attacking zangfu organs directly...OR... • deficiency of yang qi.
What is an Interior Heat Syndrome?	Group of s/sx caused by: • exogenous pathogens transmitted to the interior and changing into heat...OR... • heat pathogens directly attacking the zangfu organs.
What 2 types of heat syndromes can you have with Interior Heat Syndrome?	• Interior Xu (Deficient) Heat Syndrome • Interior Shi (Excess) Heat Syndrome
What are the definitive symptoms that mark True cold when False Heat signs are present?	• Thirsty for warm drinks, no dry throat • Wants body covering • Body feels cold • Loose stools • Clear, profuse urine • Pale tongue, white moist fur

What are the false signs in True Heat, False Cold?	• Pale face • Cold limbs
What are the false signs in True Cold, False Heat?	• Thirsty • Red face • Hot limbs
What information do the principles of Deficiency and Excess give in the Eight Principle Theory?	Relative strength of pathogens and anti-pathogenic Qi
What 2 things can you determine once you know the relative strength of pathogens vs anti-pathogenic Qi (i.e., 60%:40%)?	1. determination of the prognosis 2. determination of proper treatment
Which specific deficiency does Deficiency refer to in this case?	Zheng or Correct Qi, which is all of your qi and therefore your ability to resist attacking Evils.

Eight Principles Charts

Use these charts to compare interior and exterior and to help you understand the differences between them.

A bit of a teaching moment: I have already introduced the word "xu" for deficiency. Here's another: "shi" means excess. I've used this below because there is so much information packed into such a small space.

EXTERIOR/INTERIOR

	Exterior	Interior
Definition	Group of pathological conditions resulting from invasion of superficial portion of the body by exogenous pathogens	Pathological conditions resulting from one of two things: • Transmission of exogenous pathogenic factors to the interior of the body to affect the Zangfu organs • **OR** from functional disturbances to the Zangfu organs

	Exterior	Interior
What it tells you:	Location and stage of a disease (depth of a disease and direction the disease is developing toward—out to in, or in to out.)	Location and stage of a disease (depth of a disease and direction the disease is developing toward—out to in, or in to out.)
Locations	Superficial portions: Skin, hair, muscles, interspaces between, superficial portions of meridians and collaterals	Interior: Five zang and six fu organs
Natures	• Sudden onset • Short duration • Early stage of exogenous disease	• Chronic • Longer duration • Middle or late stage of disease

Causes	Invasion of exogenous pathogenic factors	• Transmission of a persistent pathogen from exterior to interior to invade Zangfu organs
		• Direct attack on Zangfu organs by exogenous pathogens
		• Lifestyle factors which affect Zangfu organs directly leading to functional disturbances such as:
		  o Drastic emotional changes
		  o Improper diet
		  o Overstrain and stress

	Exterior	Interior
Chief Manifestations	• Fever simultaneous to chill • Aversion and intolerance to cold, wind, chill • Pain in the limbs • Sweating or not, depending on whether heat or cold is coupled with this. • Thin white tongue coat • Superficial pulse	• High fever • No aversion to cold • Irritability, delirium, coma • Vomiting • Thirst • Either constipation or diarrhea • Tongue: yellow fur (May range from yellow to black, slippery to greasy, body may be purple, pale, trembling, deviated, etc. • Pulse: deep, slippery, wiry, choppy
Accomp. s/sx	• Headache • general aching • nasal obstrx/dischg • sneezing • coughing	
Clinical manifest-ations	• Exterior cold syndrome • Exterior heat syndrome • Exterior shi syndrome • Exterior xu syndrome	• Interior cold syndrome • Interior heat syndrome • Interior shi syndrome • Interior xu syndrome

Differentiation	• Fever
	
	• Thin white coat
	• Superficial pulse
		• Fever
		  o With no aversion to cold…*OR*…
		    No fever + aversion to cold
		• Varies
		• Deep pulse

	Cold	Heat
Definition	Pathological conditions resulting from: • Exposure to exogenous pathogenic cold *-or-* • Deficiency of Yang in interior of body	Pathological conditions resulting from: • Invasion of exogenous pathogenic heat *-or-* • Deficiency of Yin in the interior of the body
What it tells you:	Nature and stage of a disease	Nature and stage of a disease
Locations	Exterior or interior	Exterior or interior
Natures	• Belongs to Yin • Duration: long (int), short (ext)	• Belongs to Yang • Acute/urgent nature if caused by exogenous heat • Chronic if caused by deficiency (of yin, yang, qi, blood) • Duration: long (int), short (ext)

Chief Manifest ations (Sympto ms)	• Aversion to cold, pref for warmth
	• No thirst
	• Pallor
	• Cold limbs
	• Loose stools
	• Clear, profuse urine
	• Tongue: pale, white moist or greasy coat
	• Pulse: slow or tense
	• Tasteless/bland taste in mouth
		• Fever, pref for coolness
		• Thirst, pref cold drink
		• Redness of face/eyes
		• Hot limbs
		• Spirit:
		  o Irritability
		  o Restlessness
		• Dry stools or constipation
		• Urine: dark yellow, scanty, reddish
		• Tongue: red w/yellow and/or dry coat
		• Pulse: rapid

Clinical Manifest ations	• Exterior cold • Interior cold • Shi cold • Xu cold	• Exterior heat • Interior heat • Shi heat • Xu heat

Side by side s/sx comparison of Cold to Heat		
	Cold	**Heat**
Cold/ heat	Aversion to cold, prefer heat	Aversion to heat, prefer cold
Thirst	No	Yes, wants cold drinks
Face	Pale	Red
Limbs	Cold	Hot
Stools	Loose	Dry
Urine	Profuse, clear	Scanty, reddish, dark
Tongue	Pale with white and greasy coat	Red with yellow coat
Pulse	Slow and tight	Fast

TRUE/FALSE HEAT AND COLD

	True Heat + False Cold	**True Cold + False Heat**
Thirst	Yes, wants cold	Yes, wants warm
Covering	No	Yes
Face	Pale	Red
Body feels	Hot	Cold
Throat	Dry	Not dry
Limbs	Cold	Hot
Stools	Dry	Loose
Urine	Scanty, reddish	Profuse, clear
Tongue	Deep red, dry yellow coating	Pale, white moist fur
Pulse	Forceful, deep	Large, weak

INTERIOR XU AND SHI (EXCESS) COLD SYNDROMES

	Int Xu Cold	**Int Shi Cold**
Limb temp	Cold	Cold, prefers warmth
Face complex	Pale	Pale
Ab pain	Cold pain, better with pressure	Pain, worse with pressure
Stool	Loose	Loose
Urine	Clear, profuse	Clear, normal volume

Taste?		Bland
Tongue	Pale	Pale w/white coat
Pulse	Deep, slow, weak	Deep, slow, tight
Fatigue	Yes	---
SOB	Yes	----

COMPARISON: EXTERIOR COLD, HEAT, DEFICIENCY, EXCESS

	Ext Cold	Ext Heat	Ext Xu	Ext Shi
Aversions	Strong, to cold	Slight: wind and cold	Wind	
Fever	Mild	Severe	Mild	Mild
Chills	Severe	Mild	Mild	Severe
Pain	General aching	Headache	Headache Stiff neck	Headache Body pain
Sweating	No	Yes	Spontaneous	No
Thirst	No	Yes Slight + dry sensation in mouth	No	No
Tongue	Light/mild red	Red tip and edges	Pale	Mild red
Coating	Thin white moist	Thin yellow	Thin or none	Thin and white
Pulse	Floating and tight (superficial, tense)	Floating and rapid	Floating, thin, weak	Floating, strong Floating tight
Other			• Pale face • SOB • Dyspnea w/exertion • Catch cold easy • Poor appetite • Loose stool	

COMPARISON: INTERIOR COLD, HEAT, XU, SHI

	Internal cold	Internal Heat	Internal Xu	Internal Shi
Aversions	Cold, pref heat			
Fever		High		High
Chills				
Pain	Abdominal			
Sweating				
Thirst	No	Yes		
Complexion		Red eyes, lips		
Tongue		Red	Pale, swollen	
Coating	White			Yellow, old fur
Pulse	Deep, slow	Deep, fast	Deep, weak	
Stool	Loose			Constipation
Urine	Clear	Yellow, red		
Other	Cold limbs	Irritable	• Lassitude • Dizziness • Palpitation • Low voice • Less talking • Poor appetite	• Mental restlessness • Hoarse breathing

DEFICIENCY/EXCESS

	S/sx	Possible causes/notes
Body Condition	Emaciation	
Facial Complexion	Pallor	Qi xu Blood xu Yang xu
Demeanor	Listlessness	
Level of Energy	Lassitude	
Breathing	Feeble Shortness of Breath	Lung Qi Xu Zong Qi Xu

Diagnostics of Chinese Medicine:
Symptom Analysis and Syndrome Differentiation

	S/sx	Possible causes/notes
Speech/voice	Dislike of speaking	Lung Qi Xu Zong Qi Xu
Heart	Palpitations	Heart Qi Xu Zong Qi Xu
	Insomnia	Heart Qi Xu Heart Blood Xu
	Poor memory	Heart Blood Xu Short term = Heart Long term = Kidney
Sweating	Spontaneous	Qi Xu Yin Xu Yang Xu
	Night Sweating	Qi Xu Yin Xu Yang Xu
Nocturnal...	Emissions	Yin Xu Yang Xu Qi Xu
	Enuresis (*bed wetting*)	Kidney Qi Xu
Pain	Pain alleviated by pressure	Deficiency of x (Xu loves pressure)
Tremors	Yes	Liver x deficiency *Can also be excess such as external wind invasion or internal rising liver yang/fire, etc.*
Tongue	Dry Little coating No coating	Yin xu Body fluid xu Blood xu
Pulse	Of appropriate deficiency type	

YIN XU SYNDROMES

Can be many different types of Yin xu syndromes:
Lv, Ht Yin, Body Fluids, etc.

S/sx Affects:	S/sx	Probable cause(s) / Notes
Body condition	Emaciation	Yin xu
Eye	Dry	Liver yin xu
	Blurry	Liver blood xu
Fever	Afternoon fever	Yin xu
	Heat in palms and soles	Yin xu
Facial complexion	Red in zygomatic/ malar area	Yin loss and blood loss causing xu heat
Sweating	Night sweats	Yin xu
Throat and Mouth	Dryness	Yin xu Body fluid xu
Urine	Yellow (darkish)	Yin xu/yang relatively too much
Stool	Dry	Yin xu
Tongue	Red w/ little coating	
Pulse	Thready and rapid	Thready due to xu Rapid due to xu heat

YANG DEFICIENCY SYNDROMES

Yang xu usually preceded by Qi xu.

	S/sx	Notes or possible causes
Chills and fever	Chills	
Limbs	Cold	
Demeanor	Listless	Cold brings sluggishness in body and mind
Energy level	Lassitude	
Sweat	Spontaneous sweating	• Yin (body fluid) + Yang (Wei Qi) = sweat • Spontaneous sweating = Yang Qi xu (wei) cannot ctrl sweat pores, so fluids leak out.

Diagnostics of Chinese Medicine:
Symptom Analysis and Syndrome Differentiation

Thirst	None	Meaning: body fluid enough or not too much heat
Urine	Clear, increase in volume	
Stools	Loose, often with diarrhea early in the morning around 5am	
Tongue	Pale, white coating	
Pulse	Deep, weak, slow	Deep = interior Weak = xu Slow = cold

QI XU SYNDROMES

Usually precedes Yang xu

	S/sx	Notes or possible causes
Energy level	Fatigue Lassitude	
Breathing	Shortness of breath	
Voice	Weakness of voice	
Sweating	Spontaneous	(Wei Qi xu which can't control pores)
Tongue	Swollen, teeth marks, white fur	
Pulse	Soft, weak	Soft = Qi not powering blood Weak = xu

BLOOD XU SYNDROMES

	S/sx	Notes or possible causes
Vision	Blurry	Often = Lv Blood xu
Facial complexion	Pallor - Pale eyelids, mouth, lips, gums, nails	Blood cannot nourish the tissues
Energy level	Fatigue	Blood cannot carry Qi

	S/sx	Notes or possible causes
Memory and concentration	Poor memory Poor concentration	Blood carries and houses the Shen. Without it, cannot remember or concentrate. Blood xu especially affects the heart
Menses	Irregular menstruation	Insufficient blood for this
Other	Dizziness	Cannot carry clear Yang to head
Tongue	Pale with white coating	
Pulse	Weak and soft	Weak = xu Soft = insufficient Blood volume or quality

SHI (EXCESS) SYNDROMES

Syndromes of excess refer to pathological conditions in which:
1. The pathogenic factor is hyperactive
2. The antipathogenic Qi remains strong

Reasons for excess:
1. External evil attacking
2. dysfunction of internal organs

General S/sx of Excess Syndromes

	S/sx	Notes or possible causes
Demeanor	Agitation	
Voice	Loud or sonorous	
Breathing	Coarse	
Chest/abdomen	Distention and fullness	
Pain	Pain aggravated by pressure	
Bowels	Constipation Tenesmus	Straining, urgent, painful. Feels incomplete, often with burning. Damp heat is the problem. Often seen in IBS.

Urine	Dysuria	
Tongue	Thick and sticky coating	
Pulse	Excess type pulses	

EXTERIOR/INTERIOR, COLD/HEAT, XU/SHI COMBINATIONS

		Exterior/Interior + Cold/Heat + Xu/Shi (Excess) S/sx
Exterior	Cold	<ul><li>Chills greater than fever</li><li>Bland taste in mouth</li><li>Thirst: No thirst</li><li>Tongue: thin white coating</li><li>Pulse: superficial and tight</li></ul>
	Heat	<ul><li>Fever greater than chills</li><li>Thirst: Slight</li><li>Tongue: red sides and tip with thin yellow coating</li><li>Pulse: floating/superficial and rapid/fast</li></ul>
	Xu	<ul><li>Pain/stiffness:<ul><li>Headache</li><li>Stiff neck</li><li>Aversion to wind</li></ul></li><li>Fever: yes</li><li>Sweating: yes</li><li>Pulse: floating, slowed down</li></ul>
		<ul><li>Sweating: Frequently, spontaneous</li><li>Immunity: Catches cold easily</li><li>Face: pale</li><li>Breath:<ul><li>Shortness of breath</li><li>Dyspnea with exertion</li></ul></li><li>Energy: fatigued</li><li>Appetite: poor</li><li>Loose stool</li><li>Tongue: pale</li><li>Pulse: thin, weak</li></ul>

Exterior/Interior + Cold/Heat + Xu/Shi (Excess) S/sx			
	Excess (Shi)	<ul><li>Pain:<ul><li>Headache</li><li>Body pain</li></ul></li><li>Sweating: none</li><li>Pulse: Floating and tight</li></ul>	
Interior	Xu	Heat	<ul><li>Facial compl: malar flush</li><li>Body type: thin</li><li>Sweating: night sweat</li><li>Fever: palm and sole fever (5 palm heat)</li><li>Thirst: thirst with dry throat</li><li>Tongue: red with less coating</li><li>Pulse: thin and fast</li></ul>
		Cold	<ul><li>Facial compl: pale</li><li>Pain: cold pain, better with pressure</li><li>Stool: loose</li><li>Urine: profuse and clear</li><li>Energy: fatigue</li><li>Breathing: shortness of breath</li><li>Limbs: cold</li><li>Tongue: pale</li><li>Pulse: deep, weak and slow</li></ul>
	Excess (shi)	Cold	<ul><li>Facial compl: pale</li><li>Pain: abdominal pain, worse with pressure</li><li>Stool: loose</li><li>Urine: clear</li><li>Mouth: bland taste with profuse saliva</li><li>Limbs: cold, preference for warmth</li><li>Tongue: pale with white fur</li><li>Pulse: deep, slow, tight</li></ul>

Diagnostics of Chinese Medicine:
Symptom Analysis and Syndrome Differentiation

Exterior/Interior + Cold/Heat + Xu/Shi (Excess) S/sx			
		Heat	• Fever: high, preference for cold drink • Facial complexion: red face and eyes • Spirit: ○ Irritability ○ Delirium • Abdominal distension, worse with pressure • Stool: constipation • Urine: scanty, red • Tongue: red with yellow, dry coating • Pulse: flooding, slippery, fast

YIN AND YANG COLLAPSE

		Yin collapse	Yang collapse	
Sweating		Sticky, hot, salty taste	Profuse, cold, no taste	
Cold/heat		Fever in body, warm limbs	Cold body and limbs	
Breathing		SOB	Weak	
Spirit		Irritable, restless	Listless	
Thirst		Yes, cold drink	No, possible want of warm drink	
Tongue		Red, dry	Pale, moist	
Pulse		Rapid, weak	Very weak	
		S/sx	Tongue	Pulse
Y A N G	Ext.	• Aversion to cold • Fever • Aching in head and body	Thin white or yellow coat	Floating
	Heat	• Fever • Thirst with pref for cold drink • Flushed face, red eyes • Urine: scanty, yellow • Stool: constipation	Red body, yellow coat	Rapid

	Shi	• Hyperactive Breathing: hoarse • Pain: pain, fullness in abdomen/chest, worse with touch • Stool: dry Urination: difficult	Thick and greasy coat	Solid
Y I N	Int	Same as syndromes of excess and deficiency.	Thick	Deep
	Cold	• Aversion to cold, likes warmth • Pale face • Cold limbs • Urine: clear • Stool: loose	Pale body, white-moist coat	Slow
	Xu	• Pale face • Lassitude • Pain: dull • Palpitations • Weakness • Spontaneous sweating • Likes touch • Shortness of breath • Thin body	Little fur	Thin

Diagnostics of Chinese Medicine:
Symptom Analysis and Syndrome Differentiation

SECTION 2
Zangfu Diagnostic Model

Though most statistics seem to suggest that people seek out acupuncture and Chinese medical treatment for pain, I found that in my clinic it was about 50-50. About half of my patients were mostly coming for pain, and the rest were coming for stress, anxiety and/or depression, diabetes control, swollen feet and legs, fibromyalgia, insomnia, and more.

That means that at least half of my job relied heavily on Zangfu diagnosis methods. What I'm saying is it's important. It's also heavily tested on your boards. And I'm not just talking about the tests on acupuncture and foundations. I mean even the herbal board. If you can't diagnose using the Zangfu diagnostic model, passing that board is impossible.

That's why we are heavily emphasizing it in this book. It's the concrete foundation that supports a great deal of your education!

Two big things to know about the chapters in this section:

- Pay particular **attention to anything that is bolded.**

- I've also included the definitive s/sx charts for each of the Zangfu. This following symbol ✋ is an hallmark sign/symptom - this particular sign or symptom is definitive for dysfunction in this particular Zang or Fu organ. So when you see this: ✋…memorize it!

This is where it gets good, folks. Now you can move past simply looking at your families' and friends' tongues and pulses and *really* start diagnosing them all the time!

Yeah, we all do it for the first couple of years. Every time someone yawned or laughed I was secretly doing tongue diagnosis.

STUDY AND CLINICAL TREATMENT SUGGESTION

Let me insert a strong suggestion here. Create charts and comparisons for each of the Zangfu syndromes as well as for the combination syndromes.

Do this as you study each of the Zangfu organ syndromes. Here's why:

- **Learning**
  I used to provide these for you, but I think it's imperative that you create your own so that you learn the better. It's one thing to read someone elses's notes, but it's quite another to write it yourself. When you write it yourself, you incorporate more of your senses and thus more of your brain. You'll make stronger pathways to the information by doing it yourself.

- **Clinical Use**
  I not only learned the material better by doing my charts, but I laminated them and took them with me to clinic. They were super helpful in student clinic. As a matter of fact, I still refer back to them once in a while.

Creating these charts will also help you answer the study questions at the end of each chapter.

Here's a sample of what mine look like:

Heart Deficiency (Xu) Syndromes

Most common heart symptoms:

palpitation, shortness of breath worse with exertion, spontaneous sweating, pale tongue with white coat.

Heart Qi Xu	☙Palpitation
	Shortness of breath, worse with exertion also termed: "Oppression in the chest aggrivated by movement"
	Spontaneous sweating
	Listlessness
	Lassitude
	Tongue: Pale body with white coat
	Pulse: Thready and weak or irregular
Heart Yang Xu	Palpitation
	Shortness of breath, worse on exertion
	Spontaneous sweating
	☙Chills
	☙Cold Limbs
	Tongue: Pale, swollen body with slippery coating Alt: Pale, swollen body with purplish dark tongue, white slippery coating
	Pulse: Deep, weak, slow
Heart Blood Xu	☙Palpitation
	☙Insomnia
	☙Dream-disturbed sleep
	Poor memory, poor concentration
	Pallor (pale face)
	Pale lips
	Dizziness
	Vertigo
	Tongue: Pale body
	Pulse: thready, weak

This page intentionally left blank.

Diagnostics of Chinese Medicine:
Symptom Analysis and Syndrome Differentiation

CHAPTER 6
Heart and Small Intestine

The Heart (the Emperor in Chinese Medicine), joy, smiling, and laughing are all related according to the Five Element associations. This chapter will cover the common s/sx of various forms of Heart imbalances and disease. Here's what you will learn about:

- Heart Yin xu
- Heart Blood xu
- Heart fire flaring up
- Phlegm fire disturbing the Heart
- Heart heat transmitting to Small Intestine

And speaking of Small Intestine, you'll notice that there's not a lot of chat about the Yang organs.

If you remember back to your foundations studies, we talked about the Heart's role in the Zangfu pantheon. A quick review:

Zangfu Heart things:	Brief discussion
Heart governs Blood	Any kind of heat in the Blood will disturb the Heart, often resulting in poor sleep
Controls the Blood vessels	
Houses the mind	The Shen is rooted in and rests in the Blood, but it's home is the Heart. Heart fire will heat the Blood and disturb the Shen. Many kinds of mental illnesses are linked to this.
Heart manifests in the complexion	A very red face might indicate Heart problems.
Heart is related to Joy	Joy is awesome. Too much joy is mania. Not so good.
Heart opens to the tongue	Patient talks like mad and won't stop? Could be a Heart thing.

Heart controls sweating	Pay attention to feel of skin when you shake hands. Dry skin on the dorsal side + cold/wet palm could indicate Heart disease. Sweaty hands, especially when slightly nervous can be related to Heart qi's inability to control the fluids.
Heart loathes heat	Heart fire leads to insomnia because it damages the Body Fluids and thus the Blood.

Differentiation of Heart Dysfunction

First, let me just say that a "heart problem" in Chinese medicine can be very different from a "heart problem" in western medicine. That said, our version of "heart dysfunction" could very well be the precursor for biomedical cardiac problems.

I mention this because patients can get really freaked out if you tell them you detected a heart problem! They are thinking Grey's Anatomy and "Holy crap, am I going to have a heart attack?!" Be careful of your wording. Educate your patients on the difference.

Moving on.

HEART XU SYNDROMES

Differentiation of Heart dysfunction per Chinese medicine means that first you will determine whether there is deficiency or excess.

Deficient Heart Syndromes	Excess Heart Syndromes
Heart Qi xu	Heart fire flaring up
Heart Yang xu	Phlegm fire disturbing the Heart
Heart Blood xu	Stagnation of Heart Blood
Heart Yin xu	

Remember, the symbol ✋ means it's a very important or hallmark s/sx of the syndrome! **Commit it to memory!**

Diagnostics of Chinese Medicine:
Symptom Analysis and Syndrome Differentiation

Heart Qi Xu

	S/sx	Notes
🖐	Palpitations	The main and most common symptom of heart syndromes
🖐	Shortness of breath (SOB), worse with exertion	• Qi xu – lung can be related. • You're thinking Lung, but Heart and Lung are so closely tied that one affects the other. • Any time a symptom is worse on exertion think Qi xu. • Oppression in the chest which is aggrivated by movement is another way to say this.
	Spontaneous sweating	Not night sweats, but plain old spontaneous sweating
	Listlessness	Indicates Qi xu
	Lassitude	
	Tongue: pale body with white coating	Pale body indicates either Qi or Yang. White coating could be normal
	Pulse: Thready, weak, irregular	Heart Qi xu often manifests as abrupt, knotted or intermittent/irregular pulses.

The most common s/sx for Heart Qi xu are:
- Palpitations
- SOB
- Spontaneous sweating
- Pale tongue with a white coat.

Heart Yang Xu

These are very similar symptoms to those above. Yang deficiency is a Qi deficiency plus (deficient) cold. Without the fire of Yang, the water in the body will not circulate properly, but will gather and sit, causing the water retention (edema) signs you see below.

	S/sx	Notes
	Palpitations	Same discussion as Heart Qi xu above.
	Shortness of breath, worse with exertion	
	Spontaneous sweating	
✋	Chills	Definitely different from Heart Qi xu.
✋	Cold limbs	
	Tongue: pale swollen body, slippery coating	Swollen body with the slippery coat means the body is more watery and colder due to the yang deficiency.
	Pulse: Deep, weak, slow	Cold from yang xu (slow), deep because it's been around longer and the condition is chronic, weak due to deficiency.

Differences between Heart Qi def and Heart Yang def.

Some of the s/sx are the same (palpitations, SOB, worse with exertion, spontaneous sweating), but look at the differences so you can tell the difference between them.

Heart Qi xu	Heart Yang xu
--	Chills
--	Cold limbs
Pale tongue, white coat	Pale swollen tongue or dark purplish tongue, slippery white coat
Weak pulse	Deep, weak, slow

It's the cold that makes the difference. The cold makes water movement sluggish in the body, hence the swollen tongue, slippery coating, and slow pulse for Heart Yang xu.

Heart Yang Collapse

The Yang of the Heart can be so depleted that it collapses. This could be the case in severe blood loss.

Signs and symptoms include sudden, profuse cold sweat, cold limbs, feeble respiration, pale face, purple lips, unclear mind or coma. The tongue could be pale, or purple and the coat will have a watery look. The pulse will be feeble.

Heart Blood Xu

	S/sx	Notes
🖐	Palpitations	The main and most common symptom of heart syndromes
🖐	Insomnia	Normally Qi (yang) nourishes blood (yin) when you are sleeping. If the Blood cannot hold the Qi →insomnia.
🖐	Dream disturbed sleep	Due to heat in blood disturbing the blood. Dreaming is due to disturbed shen…why is it disturbed?
	Poor memory	Short term memory is controlled by the heart, so poor short term memory is the result of a heart blood deficiency and generally comes along with poor concentration. Long term memory, however, is kidney related.
	Pale face/pallor	Can be caused by Yang, Qi, Blood xu's and/or Cold.
	Pale lips	
	Dizziness	While wind can cause dizziness, Blood/Yin xu generates this wind. Malnutrition can cause Blood xu (look for itching with this too). Anemia can cause dizziness as well as vertigo.
	Vertigo	See dizziness. And yes, there is a subtle difference between the two.
	Tongue: Pale body	Shows Blood xu
	Pulse: Thin/thready, weak	Thin/thread is the poor Blood volume. Weak is a general xu s/sx.

Heart Yin Xu

Heat signs are the key difference between Heart Blood xu and Heart Yin xu!

	S/sx	Notes
✋	Palpitations	The main and most common symptom of heart syndromes
✋	Insomnia	See Heart Blood xu
✋	Dream disturbed sleep	See Heart Blood xu
	Mental restlessness	Deficient heat symptom
	Red zygomatic region of face	Just the cheekbone area
	Dryness of mouth	Xu heat burning fluids
✋	Five palm heat, tidal fever	Deficient heat symptom
✋	Night sweats	Not the same as spontaneous sweating! Xu heat sign
✋	Tongue: Red body with dry look, less to no coating	May also have cracks on the tongue. Refer back to the tongue diagnosis section in the previous book for Yin xu tongue coatings.[7]
✋	Pulse: Thready, rapid	See Yin xu pulses in previous book.[8]

Look at what Heart Blood and Heart Yin deficiencies have in common: palpitations, insomnia, dream disturbed sleep.

And look at what is different. Blood xu has memory problems, pale features, vertigo and dizziness. Yin xu has so many heat signs.

---

[7] *Diagnostic Skills in Chinese Medicine – Book 1: The Four Diagnostic Skills* (ISBN: 1096340577), available on Amazon.com in both digital and paperback format.
[8] Ibid.

Heart Fire Flaring Upward

This is the first of three excess conditions that can affect the Heart. This patient could have palpitations, but they don't make the hit list of the most frequent symptoms. This particular syndrome might be a little less obvious than the previous ones. Notice that there are no 🖐 signs or symptoms for this one. Also notice how much stronger the heat signs are than in Heart Yin xu.

S/sx	Notes
Mental restlessness or irritability	Much stronger than that of Heart Yin xu Irritability would indicate that Liver fire was also in the mix for that patient.
Insomnia	More severe than in Heart Yin xu.
Red face	Not just the cheeks – the whole face.
Thirst	Heat burning body fluids
Ulceration and pain of the mouth and/or tongue	Heart opens to the tongue. Fire will flare upwards causing mouth and tongue ulcers as well as painful, swollen tastebuds. (To clear the heart fire, use Dao Chi San formula.)
Hot/dark urine, possibly hesitant and/or painful urination	Hesitation is due to damp heat in the lower jiao. Pain is heat in the lower jiao. Hot/dark urine is a sign of heat
Tongue: red body	
Pulse: rapid	

I'm sure you've noticed differences in wording in Chinese medicine writings, case studies, and charts by now. You might find the wording for Heart Fire symptoms that look like the mini list below, but the meaning is the same.:

Patient reports being irritable, has insomnia and mind won't settle down. Has strong thirst, wants cool or cold drinks. Has pain upon urination, color is dark yellow, urinates frequently. Tongue is red with a yellow coating. Pulse is fast.

Irritable indicates not just mental restlessness but liver fire.

Phlegm Fire Disturbing the Heart

There's an awful lot of phlegm in this list and a whole lot of heat. My professor, Dr. Song Luo, told a story of Fan Jing Zhong Ju, an old Chinese man who lived a thousand years ago. Dr. Luo identified this guy as having phlegm fire disturbing the Heart. After taking the civil service boards man times over the course of 50 years and failing each time, he finally passed. He ran through the streets in fits of mania (over abundance of joy) celebrating most annoyingly. His friends finally told him that his wife had died (a lie, by the way) to bitch slap him back down to earth. It worked and broke the manic spell.

And that, my friends, is why the NCCAOM only lets us take the national boards a certain number of times! (probably not the real reason, but it made a fun little joke.)

S/sx	Notes
Delirium	
Capriciousness	
Laughter/crying	All of these – delirium, capriciousness, laughter/crying – indicate that the Shen is very disturbed, loose, unrooted. In TCM this grouping is called "strange". A strange disease is due mostly to phlegm.
Insomnia and restlessness	When the Heart Shen is disturbed one cannot fall asleep. This is a heat symptom.
Vertigo/dizziness	This is vertigo and dizziness with a far different cause than you saw in Heart Blood xu.
Fever	Heat symptom
Red face	Heat sign
Red eyes	Heat sign
Sound of sputum in the throat	Phlegm
Yellow sticky sputum with chest stuffiness	Yellow is heat. Sticky is damp/phlegm. Sputum is phlegm. Chest stuffiness indicates the Qi can't move due to the phlegm retention disturbing its' movement.

Tongue: red with yellow/greasy coat	Red is heat. Yellow/greasy is damp, phlegm, heat.
Pulse: slippery and rapid	Slippery indicates damp/phlegm. Rapid indicates heat/fire.

Fun brain twister:

Patient has dizziness, heavy feeling in head, suffocating sensation in chest, vomits. With just this little bit of info, what's your best differentiation guess from the choices below?

1. Excessive Liver Yang
2. Qi and Blood xu
3. Stagnant phlegm
4. Kidney Essence xu

If you answered stagnant phlegm, hurray! The vomiting is due to the phlegm in the Middle Jiao, fyi.

Heart Blood Stagnation

The major difference here is the purple tongue. When you write this in a chart, you call it "Stagnation of Heart Blood." If you translate this into western med speak, it's a myocardial infarction (heart attack).

	S/sx	Notes
	Palpitations	The main and most common symptom of heart syndromes.
✋	Cardiac pain	Stabbing or stuffy in nature in the precordial region or behind the sternum. Stagnation/stasis pain is prickly/stabbing, fixed in nature, worse at night. In Chinese med, if Blood cannot flow freely, there is pain.
✋	Tongue: purplish with purple spots	If the whole tongue is not purple, there might be purple spots or macula. Remember the admonition about people of Pakistani origin - they often have purple looking tongues as a rule and this is not a dysfunction.

	Pulse: thready, choppy, irregular	Choppy due to blood xu, blood stasis or phlegm. Irregular/abrupt pulse is fast, irregularly irregular.

SMALL INTESTINE

A quick review. The SI:

- Receives and further digests foods from stomach
- Separates the clear from the turbid
- Absorbs essential substances and part of the water from foods.
- Transmits the residue of food to the large intestine and residue of the water to the Bladder.

Excess heat in the Small Intestine

This is the big one to know. I've seen it a number of times in clinic. This is excessive heat of the Heart transferring to the Small Intestine. Remember that thing about the Heart loathing heat? It's totally true. It will off-load the heat to its coupled organ, the Small Intestine, the Hand Taiyang channel. The Small Intestine can't deal with that heat either, so using it's considerable connection with water metabolism, it passes this heat along familial connections - to the *foot* Taiyang channel, the Bladder.

Moral to this story: If you have a patient with heart fire or a lot of anxieties s/sx plus recurrent "bladder infections" and UTI s/sx that aren't ever bacterial related, think about this.

	S/sx	Notes
	Restlessness	
	Thirst	
✋	Hesitant, scanty, dark urine	Helloooooo heat! Major sign.
	Burning pain in the urinary tract	

Diagnostics of Chinese Medicine:
Symptom Analysis and Syndrome Differentiation

	Bloody urine	Too much heat in the Blood can break the blood vessels. That's called reckless bleeding. This is reckless bleeding in the Bladder.
	Tongue: red body with yellow coat	Heat, heat, heat
	Pulse: rapid	

Shen disturbances might be evident in this pattern as well, due to the heat that is still influencing the Heart.

There's an awesome classic formula for this called Dao Chi San which clears the fire from the Bladder/Heart and also calms the Heart. The Ht 8 points on the hand would also help. So would Li 11 and St 40 for clearing heat and damp heat.

Study Questions

If you haven't made your Heart Zangfu comparison charts yet, get busy.

Question	Answers
What are the most common s/sx of Heart stuff in Chinese medicine?	• Palpitations *The* big symptom of Ht stuff • Shortness of breath (SOB) • Spontaneous sweating • Pale tongue, white coat
What is the hallmark symptom of Heart Qi deficiency?	• Palpitations
What are the hallmark s/sx of Heart Yang xu that make it stand out from other Heart dysfunctions?	• Chills • Cold limbs
What are the key s/sx of a Heart Blood xu?	• Palpitations • Insomnia • Dream disturbed sleep
What are the s/sx that differentiate Heart Yin xu from Heart Blood xu?	Heat s/sx. Lots of xu heat signs in Ht Yin xu, none in Ht Blood xu
List the s/sx of Heart Yin xu	• Palpitations • Insomnia with dream disturbed sleep • Five palm heat and tidal fevers • Night sweats • Red tongue body with less to no coating • Thready, rapid pulse
What are the key s/sx of Heart Blood Stagnation?	• Cardiac pain • Purplish tongue and/or purple spots on the tongue

When chest oppression is aggravated by movement, what does that indicate?	• Qi deficiency
What the heck is lassitude and why does this s/sx matter?	• Lassitude is a lack of energy or motivation on a mental/emotional level. You might find this symptom in people who are depressed, but you'll also find it in Qi xu patients. . . . which could be the reason for the depression. • It matters because it shows that the Qi of the body is weak or is blocked in some way.
How does spontaneous sweating differ from night sweating	• Spontaneous sweating occurs any time of the day, and can result from Qi or Yang xu. No exertion required. • Night sweats are specific to sleeping – break out in a sweat at night or even when taking naps. Night sweating is linked to Yin xu.

What are the differences between Heart Qi xu and Heart Yang xu?	• Tongue:
	  o Ht Qi xu = pale tongue, white coat
	  o Ht Yang xu = pale tongue, swollen –or – purplish dark coat with slippery white coat
	• Temperature affectations More feelings of cold in Ht Yang xu – limbs will feel cold.
	• Pulse Heart Yang xu pulse is deep, weak, and slow.

What is this: Sudden profuse cold sweat, cold limbs, feeble respiration, pale face, purple lips, unclear mind or loss of consciousness, feeble pulse	Heart Yang Collapse Could be due to severe blood loss.
What are the three key s/sx of a Heart Blood xu syndrome?	• Palpitations • Insomnia • Dream disturbed sleep
Heart Yin xu also has those s/sx in the previous question. How do you tell Ht Blood xu from Ht Yin xu?	Ht yin xu has several deficient heat signs and symptoms. Ht Blood xu does not.
How is Heart Yin xu (xu heat) different from Heart Fire flaring?	• Similar s/sx, but more severe in Ht fire flaring – ulcerations in the mouth, urine affected, etc.
What are the heat s/sx in Phlegm Fire Disturbing the Heart?	• Delirium, laughing/crying • Insomnia/restlessness • Fever • Red face and red eyes • Yellow to sputum and tongue coating • Red tongue • Pulse is fast
What are the phlegm s/sx in Phlegm Fire Disturbing the Heart?	• Sound of sputum in the throat • Yellow sticky sputum • Chest stuffiness • Slippery pulse • Greasy tongue coating
What is the hallmark sign of a Small Intestine excessive heat?	• Hesitant scanty dark urine

CHAPTER 7
Lung and Large Intestine

While the Heart is the emperor, the Lung is the "hua gai", or covering, usually translated as imperial carriage roof. Like a carriage roof, the Lung covers and protects Heart. Because it is the air exchange system of the body, it comes into contact with the world before any other system. For this reason it is easily attacked by external factors and prone to cold.

The Lung's primary functions are to govern Qi and respiration, control the channels and blood vessels, diffuse and descend Qi and Body Fluids, and be the upper source of water. That upper source of water thing has to do with the dispersing and descending function. You could think of this as a kind of Qi respiration. The Lung Qi is dispersed downward first. Remember too that the Lung channel originates in the Middle Jiao and it's water connection.

The Large Intestine, the paired Fu organ, is responsible for controlling passage and conduction. It transforms waste into stool and recovers or reabsorbs fluids from this waste.

The Lung suffers from the following dysfunctions:

Deficient Lung Syndromes	Excess Lung Syndromes
Lung Qi xu	Wind cold invasion
Lung Yin xu	Wind heat invasion
	Retention of damp phlegm
	in the Lung
	Retention of pathogenic heat in
	the Lung

Cough and shortness of breath (abbreviated SOB in med speak and in patient charts) are the ✋ primary symptoms ✋ of Lung problems. The most common time to cough are upon major position changes – like waking and getting up in the morning or when you lie down at night. Moving between lying and standing disturbs the Qi and where the phlegm has settled.

Coughing is actually a protective function of the body. Phlegm is like a fly trap for pathogens. The body then attempts to cough out the phlegm and get rid of the ick.

With that in mind, when is the best time to stop a cough? Good question. You want the crud to come out, not just get stuck in there, so you really need to focus on removing the phlegm primarily and then stopping the cough secondarily. You need good communication with and observation of the patient to determine your priorities here.

DEFICIENT LUNG SYNDROMES

Lung Qi Deficiency

It's pretty common to see this one in both the asthma and the smoking patient populations.

	S/sx	Notes
🖐	Feeble cough	Very common and hallmark sign of Lung problems.
🖐	Shortness of breath, worse on exertion	Also typical in Lu problems. . . and of course you remember this from Heart Qi xu too.
	Clear, thin sputum	Lung unable to disperse Body Fluids, so up comes the sputum
	Lassitude, fatigue, listlessness	Qi xu s/sx
🖐	Low voice	
	Aversion to wind	Why? Not enough lung qi to protect from wind evil. Yin Qiao San – take this if you get slight chills, a little sore throat and fatigue to head off the wind evil. If you have fever, already too late.
	Spontaneous sweating	We've talked this to death – you know by now.

	Tongue: pale w/thin white coat	
	Pulse: weak	

Another possible sign to watch for is people who sit leaning forward. That can indicate a Lung Qi xu. When you study biomedicine you will also learn that this can be a sign of emphysema – Lung Qi xu!

For asthma patients, look for "the three hollows" upon the inhale. These are at Stomach 12 and Ren 22 – just above the collarbones and right in the center between them at the sternal notch. This is a sign of dyspnea, acute asthma attack and shortness of breath.

Chemo patients are often subject to lung problems as a result of the Yin and Qi depletion that chemo brings along.

To treat Lung problems such as those above, you could use the Lu 9 point (the Yuan source point), Lu 1, and St 36. St 36? Yes. This is a great point to generate Qi in general, which will then feed the Lung Qi. When you treat with herbs you use Huang Qi for this same reason – tonifies Middle Jiao Qi without generating   heat. Ginseng is another great herb to build Qi, but tends to be to hot to use long term.

Lung Yin Deficiency

A lot of these s/sx should look pretty familiar by now.

	S/sx	Notes
	Unproductive, dry cough	Have patient cough, listen for phlegm.
	Small amt of sticky sputum, even blood tinged sputum	Heat causes reckless bleeding in the lung – pressure in vessels increases with heat which can cause small breakages in the capillaries. Another reason you might see blood in the phlegm is with Qi xu the Spleen Qi is probably also deficient, so cannot hold

		blood in vessels.
	Dryness of mouth and throat and nose.	Lung yin xu heat leading to dryness. Cannot moisten and nourish. If it was just Body Fluid deficiency there would be no heat sx.
	Afternoon fever	Yin xu heat s/sx
	Zygomatic flush	
	Night sweats	
	Hot sensations in palms and soles	
	Tongue: red body with less coating	Very Yin xu sign
	Pulse: thready and rapid	Thready due to Yin xu, rapid due to xu heat.

Skin dryness all over the body can be a sign of Lu Yin xu, since the integument system is part of the Lung system. Smoking is a big culprit here. It burns away the moisture in the lung.

Ask about a history of tuberculosis and diabetes when you see these presentations. Both are a type of Yin deficiency. "Xiao ke" is a Chinese term for diabetes. The term means emaciation and thirst, implying yin deficient body type.

LU 9 is a great point for Lu Yin xu because it nourishes most of qi and yin. Shi hu and mai dong are the go-to herbs for Lung Yin xu.

Wind cold invasion

Remember some of this from the Eight Principles discussions?

S/sx	Notes
Cough	Shows you Lu is affected
Clear sputum	Clear part is important – shows cold not heat
Absence of thirst	
Nasal obstruction	Nasal stuffiness, i.e. – swollen passages
Watery nasal discharge	🖐 This has a little hand because this is the way you tell a cold invasion from a heat invasion in the Lung. Definitive difference.
Chills + fever, But chills > fever	Chills are always greater than fever in a cold invasion.
Itchy throat	Wind symptom – wind causes itching
No sweating	Because this is an excess
Headache	Cold constricts tissues causing the pain
Tongue: thin white coating	
Pulse: Floating and tense	Also called "superficial and tight" – same same.

If you are treating this with acupuncture you would use, in addition to other points, Li 4 + Lu 7 (which is a common pairing for expelling exterior invasions) and Li 20, which helps open the nose. Jing Feng Bai Du San is a nice herbal formula for treating wind cold invasions.

Wind Heat Invasion

S/sx	Notes
Cough	Shows you Lu is affected
Small amount of sticky yellow sputum	🖐 Heat causes it to go sticky (burns Body Fluids) and yellow (heat)
Thirst	
Sore throat	Could even be severe. Often with swelling. Both due to heat. Might also have itching.

Fever with chills Fever > chills	
Slight aversion to cold	
Headache	This time due to heat and swelling
Tongue: thin yellow coating	Thin due to exterior, yellow due to heat
Pulse: superficial, rapid	Superficial due to exterior, rapid from heat

The nasal discharge, throat s/sx, greater fever, tongue coat, pulse are the way to tell wind cold from wind heat.

There are some great treatments for wind heat – acupuncture, cupping, and herbs. Yin Qiao San is a great formula to use at the early stages of a wind heat invasion. If a patient comes to you in any later stage, you will need to jump to stronger raw herbs.

Retention of Damp Phlegm in the Lung

This is also called "accumulation of phlegm in the Lung" and it's a relatively common clinical thing to see. This pattern isn't heat yet. . . but probably will be unless it's treated correctly.

S/sx	Notes
Cough	Shows you Lu is affected
Profuse white sputum that is easy to expel	This is a damp sign. The lack of yellow shows you there is no heat at this point. (Heat makes it yellow and hard to get out.)
Gurgling sound with phlegm in the throat	Phlegm/damp sign
Fullness and stuffiness in the chest	Phlegm/damp in the lung making the chest feel too full
Tongue: pale body, greasy white coat	No yellow present
Pulse: slippery	Note that this is *not fast* and slippery!

This patient might also have nausea and vomiting if phlegm/damp is also in the Middle Jiao (which is not

Diagnostics of Chinese Medicine:
Symptom Analysis and Syndrome Differentiation

uncommon). This will cause the stomach Qi to rebel upwards.

Let's say this same set of symptoms progresses to heat. Here's what it would look like:

Phlegm Heat in the Lung

Also called "Retention of Pathogenic Heat in the Lung."

S/sx	Notes
Cough	Shows you Lu is affected
Thick yellow sputum	Probably more difficult to expel
Difficulty breathing	Phlegm and heat disturbing the Lung
Dry stool	Heat burning the fluids
Dark urine	
Tongue: red with yellow coating	
Pulse: slippery, fast(er)	

Example:

A guy walks into your student clinic with a cough. He reports that he has thick, yellow sputum and is having trouble getting his breath. Upon further questioning, you find he has a dry stool and his urine is dark. His tongue body looks red and he's got a yellow tongue coating.

This is phlegm heat retention in the Lung. Note that there is no "phlegm/damp heat" because the heat has burned off the damp and now it's phlegm heat.

LARGE INTESTINE SYNDROMES

One deficiency and two excesses to know.

Since we are talking about the colon, let's chat about constipation. Constipation is *usually* due to dry, but not always. Dry could be heat, but could also be a Body Fluid deficiency, which would cause dryness in the intestine, making it difficult to expel the stool. There's a great phrase in Chinese medicine about how constipation can be because "there's not enough water to float the boat." I love that.

Constipation patients may also report that they break into a sweat when defecating or trying to defecate. That's not because it's getting aerobic. This can indicate a Qi deficiency and thus the spontaneous sweating thing. The patient is expending even more Qi trying to poop, so the body is further taxed. Qi deficiency leading to constipation is about the body not having enough energy to move the stool through the Large Intestine. The stool then sits in the intestine and the body keeps reclaiming water from it and eventually it also gets dry.

Always ask constipation patients if they have been very sick recently or hospitalized. This can set patients up for a Qi deficiency and could even indicate a blood loss leading to Qi deficiency.

Final note about constipation chat: a patient may report they have had a cough for several weeks, then constipation later on. This is a progression of the Qi not being able to descend and eventually then affecting the large intestine.

Body Fluid Deficiency

Pretty simple s/sx, really. Remember back to your foundations stuidies about Body Fluids. The signs were lots and lots of dryness that was visible just by observing.

S/sx	Notes
Constipation	All due to dryness!
Dryness of the mouth and throat	
Dry skin, hair, lips, etc.	
Tongue: red body, little moisture, dry coat	
Pulse: thready	

Fun thing to know: you can sometimes you can treat a cough by relieving constipation. Ma Zi Ren Wan, for instance, is a formula based on a very oil little seed, huo ma ren. . . and an even more fun fact? Huo ma ren is the seed of the cannabis plant. Cannabis sativa, to be exact. The oil in the seed helps lubricate the dryness of the intestines.

(Don't let anyone tell you cannabis wasn't used in Chinese medicine in years past. This isn't the only reference, but you have to dig for them. Recently read an article about a body in western China that was interred many centuries ago with all kinds of weapons and treasures including almost two pounds of cannabis.)

Damp Heat in the Large Intestine

A lot of diarrhea (minus the Ki Yang xu and Sp xu types) are due to damp heat.

S/sx	Brief discussion
Abdominal pain, worse with pressure	Because it's an excess
Diarrhea with blood, pus, and mucus in the stool	That's pretty much the definition of dysentery. Mucus is due to the damp.
Strong odor to the stool	Common for heat in the intestines
Tenesmus	Constant feeling of needing to poop. Very typical damp heat presentation
Burning sensation in the anus	Also typical heat in the intestines symptom.
Tongue: . . . too much info, see →	Red tongue body in posterior area. Coating is yellow and greasy. If tongue is a bit dry, more heat than damp If a bit wet, more damp than heat. Could also have heavy sensations.
Pulse: slippery, rapid	

You'd typically use Li 11 for a large intestine damp heat. Add St 40 (damp) and St 37 (lower he-sea of the intestine).

Some herbal formulas to consider would be ge gen qin lian teng and bai tou wen teng. Ge gen in the first formula relaxes the muscles, while huang qin and huang lian clear the heat. It's a mild formula so it can be used for a lot of different patients. Bai tou wen teng is for damp heat in the intestines with a little bit of blood.

Damp Cold in the Large Intestine

You might see this more if you live in a colder climate, since climate outside the body is reflected within the body also.

S/sx	Brief discussion
Abdominal cold pain, worse with pressure	Definitely *not* a heat sensation. They may want warm drinks.
Sticky, watery stools with mucus	Sticky due to damp, not heat.
Light odor to stool	
Tongue: coating is white, greasy, thick	
Pulse: slippery, slow	

OK, want a couple of case studies? Yeah, I thought you might. I'm writing these out like you're probably going to see them on tests, quizzes, boards, etc. then laying out the s/sx and what those might mean in this context.

Case Study 1

Patient: Vera Wang, 34 year old female
Chief complaint: coughing x1 week
History: mild occasional cough, sinus and forehead ache, nasal stuffiness, clear nasal discharge, no thirst, aversion to wind and cold. Patient has a slight fever, tightness on the upper back and neck, lassitude, and low energy after having a baby. She has a light red tongue with a thin white coat. Her pulse is superficial and weak.

Here's how I approached case studies to sort and organize them in my mind. This is slow at first, but gets faster with time. I list out the s/sx and what they could indicate in my strange but effective mental process and then see how it all adds up. This is a very Sherlock Holmes approach.

Mild occasional cough	I'm already thinking Lung because of the cough, but not severe because it's mild….that or she's pretty deficient and her body can't resist because of that.
Sinus/forehead pain	Exterior invasions are often these kinds of head pains.
Nasal stuffiness	Some kind of exterior thing affecting the Lung.
Clear nasal discharge	I'm leaning toward cold at this point because discharge would be yellow if it was more heat related…
No thirst	Could be a cold invasion. She's not showing more s/sx that would point to damp retention or I might

	lean that way.
Aversion to wind/cold	I'm guessing by now this is a cold invasion, but let's keep looking and see what shakes out.
Slight fever	Hmmm. If heat there would be *more* fever...
Tightness in upper back/neck	Cold often affects these areas. Now it's totally looking like exterior cold.
Lassitude/low energy postpartum	Qi deficiency s/sx. So now I'm thinking exterior, deficiency, and cold.
Tongue = Light red body, thin white coat	Light red = normal Thin white coat cd be normal too...but definitely not heat
Pulse = superficial, weak	Superficial = exterior/surface Weak = xu

I'm actually less wordy than this. That's just for you guys.

So, I'm seeing a lot of exterior s/sx, a lot of Lung things, and cold s/sx. This is the primary show at the moment, but I also see a Qi and Blood deficiency postpartum that is still with her. Throw that in, add it all up and you have

- An underlying Qi and blood xu
- Invasion of the Lung by wind cold

If I was going to write this into this patient's chart I would say:
Diagnosis: Cough
Differentiation: Exterior deficiency wind cold invasion

Well. That's the way my professors usually expressed it. I would probably say: "exterior wind cold invasion with underlying Qi xu." Cuz I'm a rebel like that.

That's a combination of an excess (wind cold attacking the Lung) and a deficiency (Qi and Blood xu). That means your task would be to 1) expel the wind cold and 2) tonify the Qi and Blood generally and tonify the Lung Qi specifically.

Once you deal with that wind/cold invasion with something like the Jing Fang Bai Du San formula you could put this nice lady on Ba Zhen Tang.* Ba Zhen Tang is also called Women's Eight Precious. It tonifies both Qi and Blood. I'd do a custom formula and add some Huang Qi to help with both the Lung and Spleen Qi.

(Note that there is also a formula called Ba *Zheng* Tang, but that formula is for UTI like symptoms with damp and heat in the Bladder.)

Case Study 2

Eduardo, 65 y.o. male

Chief complaint: Constipation x 3 months.

History: has a bowel movement once every 3-4 days. Stools are difficult to pass, occasionally there is a little bit of blood, are small and pebble-like in shape. Urine is darker yellow. Patient has little motivation, little energy, looks emaciated. Says he is almost always thirsty, sometimes wakes up covered in sweat, has an occasional dry cough. Past history: No hospitalizations, but had tuberculosis approximately 20 years ago.

Physical exam: You palpate the path of the large intestine on the abdomen and find the whole length of the descending colon feels tight and somewhat hard. His tongue is thin red with cracks, very little coating. The pulse is deep, thready and fast.

What's up with this guy?

Constipation x 3 months	Chronic, suggesting xu
Stool hard to pass, some blood, dry and pebbly	Dry sx for sure
Urine is darker yellow	Heat
Little motivation/energy	Xu symptom
Emaciation	Yin Xu sign

Thirst	Heat/dry
Night sweats	Yin xu
Occasional dry cough	Lung affected, dry = bf xu, xu heat
Hx of tuberculosis	This can tax the Lung heavily and often leads to a Lung yin xu
Hardness @ descending colon	Retention of stool
Tongue: thin, red, cracks, no coat	Yin xu city!
Pulse: deep, thready, fast	Deep = interior, thready = xu, fast = heat

How does all that add up to you? I'm seeing a lot of deficiency, yin deficiency s/x, and heat. Heck, the pulse alone tells the story – interior deficient heat! Boom yin xu with xu heat.

What do you do about this? Needle using reducing methods to clear the xu heat, nourish the Lung Yin, moisten the large intestine.

Want some more practice? Of course you do! Do the practice questions starting on the next page.

Practice exercises
Answer key is at the end.

1. What is indicated by this pattern: cough that produces a small amount of thick yellow sputum, thirst, sore throat, fever, slight aversion to cold, red tongue tip with thin yellow fur, floating-rapid pulse?
   a. Dry pathogens attacking the Lungs
   b. Invasion of the lungs by wind heat
   c. Retention of excessive heat in the lungs

2. Which of the following is not a clinical manifestation of Deficient Lung Qi?
   a. Feeble cough

    b. Spontaneous sweating, aversion to wind
    c. Slippery pulse

3. What is indicated by this pattern: cough with profues white sputum that is easily expectorated (spit out), pale tongue with white and greasy fur, slippery pulse?
    a. Accumulation of phlegm-damp in the lungs
    b. Wind-cold attacking the lungs
    c. Invasion of the lungs by wind heat

4. What is indicated by this pattern: cough that produces thick yellow sputum, difficult breathing, dry stools, dark urine, and red tongue with yellow fur?
    a. Accumulation of phlegm-damp in the lungs
    b. Retention of pathogenic heat in the lungs
    c. Invasion of the lungs by wind-heat

5. What is indicated by this pattern: pain in the abdomen, dysentery with mucus and pus or blood in the stools, tenesmus, a hot sensation in the anus, greasy yellow tongue fur?
    a. Damp-heat in the spleen and stomach
    b. Excessive heat in the small intestine
    c. Damp-heat in the large intestine

6. What is the main clinical manifestation of deficient body fluid in the large intestine?
    a. Pale tongue
    b. Dry stools and difficulty in defecation
    c. Dizziness

7. Have you made your s/sx charts for the Lung and Large Intestine?
    a. Yes
    b. No
    c. I've been meaning to get to that

Answer key:
1 = B, 2 = C, 3 = A, 4 = B, 5 = C, 6 = B

Question 7 should be a. Yes. Make that happen.

Study Questions

If you haven't made your Lung Zangfu comparison charts yet, get busy. (Dang, I'm pushy, aren't I?)

Question	Answers
What are the most common s/sx of a problem with the Lung?	• Cough • Shortness of breath (SOB)
There are three hallmark signs of a Lung Qi deficiency. What are they?	• Feeble cough • SOB, worse with exertion • Low (volume) voice
What is reckless bleeding and what does that do?	Reckless bleeding is the fast, more forceful movement of blood caused by heat conditions in the body. This causes capillary breakage and thus petechial, bruising.
What are the common tongue coatings you are likely to see in a Yin xu?	• Thinner coating – way less than normal. Could just be thinning in spots, depending on the organ involved. • Map coating – portions of the tongue coat looked peeled off, location dependent on organs involved. • Mirror or no coating – lack of coating.
What is a common Yin xu pulse?	Thready and thin

What is the likely differentiation for this patient? Dry skin, long term smoker, history of tuberculosis, unproductive dry cough, thready rapid pulse.	Lung Yin xu
How about this guy? Cough with thick, yellow sputum. Dude has trouble breathing. Dry stool, dark urine, red tongue with a yellow greasy looking coating?	Retention of phlegm heat in the Lung.
Why could dehydration (Body Fluid xu) cause constipation?	"Not enough water to float the boat." Insufficient moisture in the body to lubricate the intestine
What could cause dysentery type diarrhea with blood, mucus, and pus in the stools with really smelly stools?	Damp heat in the Intestines
A patient comes in with abdominal pain that feels cold, complains of sticky watery stools with what looks like mucus and that has very little odor, and she has a slippery, slow pulse. What's her differential diagnosis?	• Her diagnosis (which is always pretty close the chief complaint) is abdominal pain. • The differentiation is what you think is causing that chief complaint, which in this case is: Damp cold in the Large Intestine

This page intentionally left blank.

Diagnostics of Chinese Medicine:
Symptom Analysis and Syndrome Differentiation

CHAPTER 8
Spleen and Stomach

Once upon a time during the Jin and Yuan dynasties there were four famous doctors who created important theories that shaped Chinese medicine. Li Dong Yuan, known to friends and family as Li Gao, was one of these famous dudes. Li Dong Yuan developed a theory which stated that all problems are due to Spleen and Stomach dysfunction and this was mostly due to dumbass lifestyle choices. The name of his theory was the Spleen and Earth Theory.

Because the function of the Spleen and Stomach are critical to the proper function of the body, many syndromes and problems are related to dysfunction of the Middle Jiao. These include:
- Digestion problems of all kinds
- Wei syndrome, which includes muscle weakness, muscular atrophy (i.e. Multiple Sclerosis and other types), and wind stroke.
- Blood deficiencies, including anemia
- Bleeding problems where Spleen cannot hold the blood
- Organ prolapses due to extreme Qi deficiency
- Edema
- Weight management problems

In this chapter we will discuss five Spleen dysfunctions and four Stomach dysfunctions. Spleen is mostly about deficiency while Stomach is mostly about excess.

Deficient Spleen Syndromes	Excess Spleen Syndromes
Spleen Qi xu	Damp cold accumulation in the
Spleen Yang xu	Spleen
Spleen Qi sinking	
Spleen unable to control Blood	

Deficient Stomach Syndromes	Excess Stomach Syndromes
Stomach Yin xu	Excessive fire in Stomach
	Cold retention in Stomach
	Food retention in Stomach

SPLEEN SYNDROMES

Let's do a quick review of the Spleen's functions before we talk about dysfunctions.

Spleen's job is to:
- Govern transformation and transportation
- Control ascending of Qi
- Raise Clear Yang upwards
- Control Blood
- Control muscle and the four limbs

Now let's explore what it can look like when the Spleen can no longer do its' job effectively. You note there aren't a whole bunch of little hands 🖐 here. That's really because the hallmarks of these dysfunctions are the collection of symptoms and signs you will see repeated in the Spleen syndromes.

Regardless, **if it's bold** or has the little hand 🖐, you really need to make sure you know that.

Spleen Qi Deficiency

Ah, the core of so many problems!

	S/sx	Notes
	Sallow complexion	Indicates dampness along with the xu. Qi xu can also be pale, but usually see sallow.
✋	Lassitude	
	Dislike of speaking	
✋	Reduced appetite	Often this is the 1st symptom
✋	Gas and bloating	Qi is deficient and cannot move well. Digestion is impaired due to weakness, but so is water management in the Middle Jiao, leading to dampness and further inability to move food and qi.
	Abdominal distention worse after eating	Common symptom here. Takes a lot of Qi to digest and process food! When the Qi is already depleted, makes it even harder on the Spleen.
	Loose stools	Ascending function is impaired, so stool passes too quickly without being held for best digestion of food and for moisture reabsorption.
	Tongue: pale body, white coat	
	Pulse: weak and soft	Especially in the middle right position.

You will see several of these s/sx repeated in Spleen Yang deficiency and in Spleen Qi sinking because both of those are advanced versions of Spleen Qi deficiency.

There are some excellent effective methods of treating Spleen Qi problems, but I think the best is nutritive therapy. This is a lifestyle problem. Fix the lifestyle. Unfortunately, a lot of people simply won't, so herbs are your next best step. You can use ren shen (ginseng) to tonify Qi, but this requires regular monitoring. Ginseng can generate fire which can burn off Body Fluids and further damage the body. Another option is huang qi, astragulus. Si Jun Zi Tang, also called Four Gentlemen, is a very good formula to tonify Spleen Qi. There are some variations of this, like Liu Jun Zi Tang (Six Gentlemen) which also resolve damp.

Yu Ping Feng San, also called Jade Screen is a tonifying formula often used prior to allergy season. If taken starting about two months prior to the season that generally affects your patient, can mitigate allergy symptoms. It is gentle enough to be taken year round.

Stomach 36 is a good acupuncture point to tonify the Spleen and the Stomach. Add Spleen 6 and you are too cool for school. LI 10 + ST 36 is another good combination to balance upper and lower jiao. UB 20 will also help.

Spleen Yang Deficiency

A Spleen Yang xu differs from Spleen xu in that xu cold symptoms are added. This indicates a progression of badness from Spleen Qi deficiency to Spleen Yang deficiency.

	S/sx	Notes
	Pae and sallow complexion	Qi and yang xu + cold + Blood xu.
	Lassitude	All the same as in Spleen Qi xu
	Dislike of speaking	
	Reduced appetite	
	Abdominal distention worse after eating	
	Loose stools	
	Cold in the limbs	Different from Sp Qi xu!
	Dull abdominal pain, better with warmth/pressure	Shows the deficiency and the cold in the Middle Jiao

	Tongue: pale swollen body, white slippery coat	Added swollen tongue body and slippery coating – both damp and cold
	Pulse: deep, weak and slow	Deep indicates disease going deeper, slow indicates addition of cold.

Again, lifestyle therapy is the best choice. I'd add in some medical qigong to tonify Spleen. Check out the Six Healing Sounds qigong to help with organ dysfunction too.

Kitchen herbal therapy could consist of a little bit of ginger and brown sugar cooked together with the white parts of the scallion. The patient takes just a little of this at a time. The sugar is good for the Spleen in small doses, ginger is great for digestion and warming and so are the scallions. Come to think of it, this sounds like part of a marinade.

Moxibustion at Stomach 36 and Ren 12 are excellent tonification and warming therapies as well.

Spleen Qi Sinking

This chronic and severe situation is another progression from Spleen Qi deficiency. Note the similar s/sx compared to Spleen Qi xu and the addition of the heaviness and sinking s/sx.

	S/sx	Notes
	Sallow complexion	
	Lassitude, extreme fatigue	Like Spleen Qi xu, but more progressed.
	Low voice, dislike of speaking	
	Reduced appetite	Often this is the 1st symptom
	Dizziness	Spleen cannot ascend clear Yang
	Heavy, distending sensation in abdomen, worse after meals.	Might also be called a "bearing down" sensation. This is due to the Spleen Qi sinking – no longer able to lift and hold, nor to ascend Yang.

	Loose stools	
	Frequent bowel movements, even long term diarrhea	Ascending function *really* impaired. Cannot hold food or stool well.
	Heavy sensation around anus	Sinking Qi bearing down, causing heavy feeling
	Organ prolapses	Rectal prolapse, uterine prolapse, bladder prolapse, and stomach prolapse are all strong possibilities – Spleen cannot hold organs in place.
	Tongue: pale body, white coat	
	Pulse: feeble	Progression from weak to feeble

You can use the Du 20 point to lift the Qi, and Bl 20 to tonify the spleen. You can also use a moxibustion cone on a slide of ginger over the umbilicus, which is pretty amazing for this condition.

Cut a slice of fresh ginger about the thickness of a US nickel – 1-2mm – and poke 4 or 5 holes in it with a thick sewing needle (a three edged needle or lancet will do the trick too). Place it over the belly button and place a moxa cone of appropriate size on top of the slice. Burn several moxa cones over the ginger slice, changing the slice as needed, to tonify the Middle Jiao and the Qi.

Diagnostics of Chinese Medicine:
Symptom Analysis and Syndrome Differentiation

Spleen Unable to Control Blood

Notice the similarities to Spleen Qi sinking and the addition of the bleeding s/sx starting with purpura.

	S/sx	Notes
	Pale or sallow complexion	All the same as Sp Qi xu because this is an extention of that.
	Lassitude	
	Dislike of speaking	
	Reduced appetite	
	Abdominal distention worse after eating	
	Loose stools	
	Purpura	Bleeding under the skin at the capillariy level
	Bloody stools	Spleen qi sinking + unable to control blood
	Excessive menstrual flow	Spleen unable to control blood.
	Uterine bleeding	Abnormal uterine bleeding – either postpartum or during other times.
	Tongue: pale body, white coat	
	Pulse: weak and soft	Especially in the middle right position.

Herbal therapy would be excellent. From an acupuncture treatment perspective, consider using the Xi cleft points (very effective for blood) – SP 8, UB 17, SP 10. Tonify at Sp 6, St 36.

Damp Cold Accumulation in the Spleen

This is the only excess condition of the Spleen in the list. But this too can stem from Spleen Qi xu.

	S/sx	Notes
	Fullness and cold sensations in epigastria and abdomen	

	Poor appetite	
	Sticky saliva	This isn't phlegm – it's thickened saliva and indicates dampness.
	Nausea	Caused by damp retention in the Middle Jiao. Seems like a stomach problem, which it is, but the root is Spleen unable to process water correctly.
	Heaviness of head and body	These sensations are caused by damp retention.
	Edema	More water metabolism problems
	Loose stools	Shows the Spleen Qi xu.
	Tongue: Pale body with greasy white coating	Greasy shows the damp. Pale shows the Qi xu underneath.
	Pulse: slow, slippery	Slow is the cold, slippery is the damp. (Compare that to Sp Yang xu – deep weak, slow pulse)

Quick version of treatment: Moxa at St 36. But there are tons more things you can do. The treatment suggestions are just to give you an idea.

STOMACH SYNDROMES

The Stomach gets more press here than most Yang organs because it is such a crucial player in the generation of Qi and in the Middle Jiao's functions. While the Spleen is responsible for lifting, the Stomach is the counterbalance, doing the descending work.

The Stomach:
- Controls receiving of food and drink
- Controls the rotting and ripening of food (creating chime in the stomach organ)
- Controls the transportation of food essence
- Controls descending of Qi

- Likes wet conditions, disliked dry and heat
  (Spleen by comparison, likes dry and heat and doesn't like having wet feet!)

Stomach has three excessive conditions and one deficiency we will talk about.

Excessive Fire in the Stomach

This is an acute disease. Compare and contrast it with the chronic deficient fire you see in the final Stomach dysfunction in this section, Stomach Yin deficiency.

	S/sx	Notes
🖐	Burning pain in the epigastric region	
	Sour regurgitation	Indicates St not descending Qi
	Thirst for cold	Heat
🖐	Voracious appetite! Easily hungry	Fire consuming resources! FYI, bulemia is treated as excessive stomach fire – uncontrollable appetite uncontrollable + repeat vomiting leads to fire s/sx.
	Foul breath	Food rots and sits too long because St not descending
	Swelling, pain, ulceration, bleeding of gums	Especially upper gums.
	Constipation	Stomach cannot descend Qi, heat burns Body Fluids
	Scanty, deeper yellow urine	Another s/sx of heat burning Body Fluids
	Tongue: red body with yellow coating	
	Pulse: rapid	

Stomach 44 is a great point for this, as it is a summary of the whole treatment process – reduce fire, promote function of stomach, stop that reckless bleeding.

Cold Retention in the Stomach

The is a relatively excessive condition. You can see the cold signs evident in this list.

	S/sx	Notes
✋	Cold and contraction type pain in Stomach, better after eating warm meals	
	Cold pain is worse in cold environment	Could be cold outside or sitting in AC or even swimming in a cold pool–either way, it's a cold environment
	No thirst	
	Prefers warmth	
	May have an aversion to touch	Excess symptom
	Possible nausea and vomiting	More like probably n/v
	Tongue: Pale body white coat	
	Pulse: slow, deep	

This is another case for moxa at St 36.

Food Retention

Pretty common in my clinical experience.

	S/sx	Notes
✋	Distention, fullness, pain in epigastrium and abdomen	Too full, Qi not moving, food rotting but not moving.
	Foul belching	Sour smell to belch.
	Anorexia	This isn't about dysfunctional weight control, but about the St not being able to process more, so don't want to eat.
	Vomiting	Qi rebellion – going up instead of down
	Tongue: slightly red body, coat is thick, sticky, curdy	Tongue could be redder – stagnation like this will generate heat. If it's been happening a while the tongue will be redder.

	Pulse: slippery	Food retention in this case. Remember from pulse diagnosis that slippery pulses are the result of flow disturbance in the pulse. Food retention and damp are two reasons for this.

Stomach Yin Deficiency

The only deficiency in the Stomach dysfunctions so far. This is empty heat in the Stomach. Compare that to the previous description of excessive fire and *know those differences!*

	S/sx	Notes
	Obscure and burning pain in the epigastric region	Not so obvious as excessive fire
	Empty and uncomfortable sensation in St	I've had patients describe it as hollow
	Hunger, but no desire to eat	Sensation from empty fire. Patient may eat tiny amounts frequently.
	Dry vomiting and hiccups	Dryness from Yin xu
	Dryness of mouth, throat	Also Yin xu
	Constipation	From the dryness when xu heat burns Body Fluids. Also, yin = moisture, so yin xu = less moisture.
	Tongue: Red body, xu coatings	Shape of the tongue body could be narrow, might have cracking across surface.
	Pulse: thready, rapid	Typical of Yin xu.

Case 1

30 yo female.
Seeking acupuncture for weight control.

History of eating uncontrollably then purging. Goes on strict diets, fasts, does vigorous exercise. Has a history of vomiting, using laxatives and diuretics to lose weight. Sometimes vomits blood and uses the bathroom frequently after meals. Suffers from depression and mood swings. Feels out of control. Swollen glands in neck and face. Has heartburn, bloating, indigestion, constipation, irregular periods, dental problems, sore throat, weakness, exhaustion, blood shot eyes. Reports a burning pain in epigastric region w/preference for cold beverages. Strong smell to her breath. Has frequent ulcers on on upper gums. Abdominal palpation is uncomfortable, doesn't like the pressure. Red tongue with yellow coat, rapid pulse.

Diagnosis is excessive Stomach fire
She's clearly a bulimia patient, but in many places you cannot say that in your charting as this is a western medical diagnosis we are not allowed to make.

Case 2

28 year old female.
Chief complaint is missed periods

Patient presents with a body weight that is not consistent for her age and build – she is at least 15% below normal weight with protruding bones visible. She has missed at least 3 consecutive periods. Has a vague burning pain and a hollow sensation in her belly. Hungry, but unwilling to eat, especially in public. Talks frequently about caloric intake. Frequent retching (dry vomit) and hiccups. Says her mouth

and throat frequently feel dry, wants cool water to sip. Frequent constipation.
Tongue is red, very little coating. Pulse is thready, rapid.

Diagnosis: Stomach Yin xu.
Is she also anorexic? Heck yeah, she is, but again, you can't put that in your charts in most places as this is a medical diagnosis, not a Chinese medical diagnosis.

Study Questions

If you haven't made your Spleen/Stomach Zangfu comparison charts yet, get busy.

Question	Answers
What are the key s/sx of a Spleen Qi xu?	• Lassitude • Reduced appetite • Gas and bloating
Spleen Yang xu looks similar to Spleen Qi xu. What are the s/sx that helps you tell one from the other?	• Cold limbs – all four • Dull abdominal pain that is better with pressure • Tongue is pale, but also swollen and has a greasy/slippery coating • Pulse is deep, slow, weak.
Which is worse: Spleen Qi xu or Spleen Qi sinking?	Spleen Qi sinking. This is a severe and advanced form of Sp Qi xu.
What are the Sp Qi sinking s/sx that make it different from Sp Qi xu?	• Heavy sensation in the abdomen that is worse after meals. • Frequent bowel movements • Heavy sensation in anus • Organ prolapse/s • Extreme fatigue, lassitude, low voice or dizziness • Feeble pulse • Pale, swollen tongue with a greasy or slippery coating
What are the s/sx that let you know a patient has Spleen Qi xu with a failure of Sp to control Blood?	• Purpura – bleeding under skin • Bloody stools • Excessive menstrual flow • Abnormal uterine bleeding

What are some of the damp s/sx in Spleen Damp Cold Accumulation?	• Poor appetite • Sticky saliva • Nausea • Heavy head and body • Edema • Greasy tongue coating • Slippery pulse
What is the key s/sx of Excessive Stomach Fire	Burning pain in the epigastric region
What kind of tongue coating can you expect to see in Food Retention?	• Thick, bean curd/tofu like coating that can be scraped off fairly easily.

Did I mention you need to be making your own charts? Because you do.

Diagnostics of Chinese Medicine:
Symptom Analysis and Syndrome Differentiation

CHAPTER 9
Liver and Gallbladder

The Liver technically located in the Middle Jiao to the right of the Stomach, but the energy of the Liver is in the Lower Jiao. Because the Liver stores Blood, it is another important organ related to sleeping. At night the Yang of the body dives into the interior, going to the Liver. A lot of patients with Liver dysfunction may go to sleep just fine, but will wake in the middle of the night around 2-3 in the morning and have difficulty getting back to sleep. If you check the bioclock, you see that is right in the middle of the period in which the Liver is at its peak.

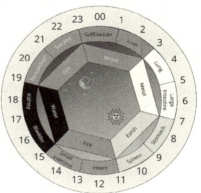

The functions of the Liver are as follows. This is just for review so you don't have to look it up.

1. Stores Blood
2. Ensures the smooth flow of Qi in the whole body and is in charge of the biorhythms. (Dysfunction of bio-rhythms in biomedicine is considered to be an endocrine disorder. Chinese medicine says the Liver is in charge of the endocrine functions.
3. Regulates blood volume in relation to rest and activity
4. Regulates menstruation
5. Moistens eyes and sinews/tendons

We are going to talk about two deficiencies and four excesses of the Liver .

Liver Deficiencies	**Liver Excesses**
Liver Yin xu	Liver Qi stagnation
Liver Blood xu	Liver fire flaring up
	Liver Yang hyperactivity
	Cold in the Liver meridian

There is one more Liver excess to talk about, Liver wind. Liver wind is an excess. The deficiencies noted above, Liver Yin xu and Liver blood xu, can generate this wind. Heat in the Liver can also generate this inner wind. We will discuss more about Liver wind after the Liver Excesses section in this chapter.

There are also two excesses of the Liver's coupled organ, the Gallbladder to know.

Gallbladder Excesses
Damp heat in the Gallbladder
Disturbance of phlegm due to Gallbladder stagnation

LIVER DEFICIENCIES

Liver Yin Deficiency

Liver Yin deficiency is the precursor to one of the excesses you will see later, Liver Yang rising. When Liver Yin is deficient the delicate balance between Liver Yin and Liver Yang is impaired. Liver Yin keeps the Yang anchored. Without sufficient Yin, Yang floats upward. That's why this is the beginning of Liver Yang rising.

Liver Yin xu can also be a precursor to Liver Blood xu, which you will see next.

	S/sx of Lv Yin xu	Notes
	Dry, itching eyes	Liver opens to the eyes. Compare this to Lv Blood xu. This is the milder of the two.
	Dizziness and vertigo	Beginning of Lv wind. Lv Yang floats free of the Yin and causes this sensation.
	Dry throat and mouth	Common yin xu s/sx
✋	Slight burning pain in the hypochondriac region	Location of pain is important – hypochondriac region is just below the rib cage at the basic level of the Liver. The slight burning pain is deficient heat.
	Shivering of the limbs	Trembling, not necessarily cold! This is another form of wind.
	Five palm heat, tidal fever, hot flashes	Common Yin xu s/sx
	Night sweating	
	Tongue: red with little to no coating	
	Pulse: wiry, thin, rapid	Thin and rapid are deficiency and heat, but wiry tells you the Lv is involved

Liver Blood Deficiency

	S/sx	Notes
✋	Blurry vision, dry eyes, night blindness	Blurry vision is a primo symptom of Lv Blood xu. Dry eyes and night vision impairment because Lv opens to the eye and without proper blood supply cannot nourish the eye. This is an advanced form of Lv Yin xu.
	Pale nails	Nails are the continuation of the tendons, which are the tissues controlled by the liver. Anemia, which shows as pale nails, is a blood deficiency problem. Dry cracking nails are other markers of this.

	Numbness of the limbs, muscle contractions, tendon and joint spams.	Blood not nourishing the tissues.
	Shivering, contractions or spasms of muscles	Another s/sx of Lv wind due to Lv Blood xu. The *Neijing* says: "Xue xu sheng feng," aka, blood deficiency generates wind. Can start as rashes and itching – wind is often accompanied by itching.
	Dizziness and vertigo	Blood deficiency causing inner wind. Anemia can cause these symptoms.
	Possible headache	Will likely be dull and empty in nature.
	Scanty menstrual flow, infertility in females	Blood deficiency means there is less blood *to* flow. Lack of nourishment due to Lv Blood xu means there is not enough nutrition to the uterine lining and it is therefore less able to support a fetus.
	Tongue: pale	Common Blood xu sign
	Pulse: thin and weak	Common Blood xu pulse.

Though Liver Blood xu can happen to anyone, it is very common for postpartum women to suffer from both Liver Blood xu and Qi xu. A common formula designed for this population is called *Ba Zhen Tang*. This is a combination of two other formulas – Si Jun Zi Tang, designed to tonify Qi, and Si Wu Tang, a Liver Blood tonification formula.

Here's a little fun exercise. Let's say a woman walks into your clinic one afternoon three months postpartum. She says she has dizziness, tinnitus, a dull and sallow complexion, she's always fatigued, and she has dry eyes and numbness in her hands.

This could be any of a number of deficiencies, but her diagnosis is Liver Blood xu. Which of the s/sx makes that clear?

If you said dry eyes, give yourself a gold star!

Liver Qi Stagnation

This is fairly common in clinic and is tied to a number of menstrual dysfunctions. It's also something that happens fairly routinely after a cholecystectomy (gallbladder removal surgery).

	S/sx	Notes
	Stress and depression	Also anxiety and depression.
	Irritability and anger	Heat generated by stagnation can cause this. Sometimes patients will report they are easy going, but their partners might report otherwise! Also, these folks may think they are easygoing because they blow up easily, which relieves the stuck Qi and makes them feel better. . . at the expense of those around them!
	Intermittent sighing for no particular reason*	Patient might not even know they are doing it. It happens when the Qi gets stuck in the chest, causing chest stuffiness. Sighing is a way to move the stuck Qi. Ren 17 is a good point for this.
	Chest stuffiness	See previous s/sx
	Epigastric and abdominal distention and pain	Liver/wood causing problems with Middle Jiao/earth. Lv/Gb meridians also cross through this area when they are moving Qi around. See diagram below.
🖐	Distending and/or wandering pain in the costal and/or hypochondriac region	You will sometimes see this referred to as "flank" pain.
	Poor appetite	Liver overacting on the MJ. Or wood overacting on earth.
	Belching	

	PMS, irregular menstruation and dysmenorrhea*	All PMS s/sx are Liver Qi stagnation. Irregular means not regular timing – might never now when the period is going to happen. Dysmenorrhea is painful menstrual. *Please note: cold pain during the period is different and due to Cold in the Lv meridian, **not** Lv Qi stagnation.*
	Distending pain in the breasts	I mention this specifically even though I already mentioned distending chest pain because it is such a common PMS sign – pain in the breasts because they feel too heavy and distended right before the period starts.
	Tongue: thin white coating, could be purplish	Though there is no real "Qi stagnation" tongue, if the patient has Qi stagnation long enough the tongue will take on a purplish cast.**
	Pulse: wiry	Especially on the left (. . . but on some patients you will feel it on the right.)

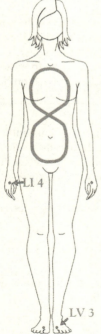

LI 4

LV 3

*The Qi circulates in a figure eight pattern through the trunk of the body. Just like in NASCAR, things slow down on the curves and speed up on the straightaways. You'll notice those slow-downs at the chest and at the lower abdomen in the drawing to the left.

Sighing is a way to move the Qi in the chest somewhat manually. Because you can't exactly sigh into the lower abdomen, the Qi gets stuck here too. Many women with PMS and dysmenorrhea feel better as soon as the bleeding starts for this reason.

Diagnostics of Chinese Medicine:
Symptom Analysis and Syndrome Differentiation

See the LI 4 and LV 3 points noted here? Together these points are called "The Four Gates" and are used in combination to treat Qi stagnation. These are very powerful points to move Qi - so powerful in fact, that they are contraindicated in pregnancy.

**One final note about that tongue. The body is an active and dynamic thing, so you could see all kinds of presentations combinations here. Using me, a Liver Qi stagnation poster child, as an example: my tongue is pale, swollen, and has teethmarks. Why? Probably because the Liver Qi stagnation is secondary to my other claim to fame, Spleen Qi deficiency with dampness. Never stake your claim on just one sign or symptom! Make sure all the evidence adds up to a good working conclusion.

Liver Qi stagnation could look like this:
> 35 y.o. woman complains of irregular and painful menstrual cycles. Sometimes she has no period at all. She has breast distention and pain the week before her period. Also has a sensation of fullness in the chest and abdomen. Sighs intermittently and deeply. When questioned, she doesn't know why she does that. Reports large dark clots in her menstrual bloods.

Liver Fire Flaring Up
The Liver and the Heart are the two Yin organs with the strongest association with fire. You actually need a firey quality to these organs, and yet you need to balance to keep them from getting too firey.

Liver fire flaring upward is an excess condition of the Liver that can be caused by something as simple as extreme anger. That could be a great reason not to consume too much news! Though "Liver fire flaring" sounds pretty alarming, this is not as severe as Liver Yang rising, as you will see in the s/sx list.

Though it *is* lower on the severity totem pole, Liver fire flaring upward can still burn the Yin of the Liver and eventually *cause* the more serious condition of Liver Yang rising. Liver fire flaring can also cause wind in the body, like an internal tornado.

Here is what Liver fire flaring upwards looks like:

	S/sx	Notes
🖐	Distending pain in the head	
	Redness, swelling, and pain in the eyes	S/sx of heat
	Bitter taste and dryness in the mouth	Heat burning the body's resources, causing both the bitter taste and the dryness.
	Burning pain in the costal and hypochondriac area	Heat symptom. Hypochondriac area, also called flanks in some texts, is where the Liver dysfunction expresses.
	Hematemesis, hemoptysis	Hematemesis is the vomiting of blood – this is Lv overacting on St. Hemoptysis is spitting up or coughing up blood – Lv insulting Lu.
	Anger, irritability	More heat symptoms
	Tongue: red body, yellow coating	
	Pulse: wiry, rapid	

The Ying Spring point of the Liver channel, Lv 2, would be a nice choice for acupuncture points to help with this.

Liver Yang Rising

Also called Liver Yang Hyperactivity in some texts and Excessive Liver Yang in others. This is an important pattern and is relatively severe. This is the natural outflow of unchecked Liver Yin deficiency!

There are actually two reasons Liver Yang can begin to rise and become excessive:

1. Excess
   Sudden extreme anger makes the Lv Yang rise. Though this is a temporary condition, it can become a repeat pattern and cause frequent problems. Anger and outrage can be quite addictive it seems.

2. Deficiency
   Liver Yin and Liver Yang must be in balance. If the Liver Yin, the anchor for Liver Yang, becomes deficient, the Liver Yang will do it's yangy thing and float upward. This takes time, so as Liver Yin deficiency gets more chronic and unchecked, the Liver Yang will tend to float upwards.

   Older people suffer from this more often than young ones do. As people age the Kidneys get more deficient, thus Water is deficient and cannot nourish the Wood element. Liver Yin and Kidney Yin xu's are often coupled, especially in the case of hypertension in older peeps. Kidney controls essence, Liver controls blood. One can generate the other and are the same source.

   Because Liver and Kidney are BFFs, a deficiency of Kidney Yin will also lead to a deficiency of Liver Yin.

S/sx	Notes
Severe dizziness and vertigo	Inner wind causes these sensations and is very strong…which is why the Shen is disturbed – see insomnia below in this table.
Headache	May be due to hypertension. These types of headaches are often a distending or throbbing pain.
Flushed face	Due to heat of Yang rising upwards
Red eyes	
Palpitations	Because of the wood/fire (Lv/Heart) mother and son relationship
Frequent irritability, agitation	Often tied to heat s/sx in the body
Insomnia w/ dream disturbed sleep	Shen is disturbed by heat – again because of the wood/fire (Lv/Ht) mother and son relationship
Soreness and weakness of the lower back and knees	This is the Kidney, Lv's bestie, also impacted by the underlying Yin xu. Lower back and knees are often affected in Kidney xu. *
Tongue: scarlet to deep red body, little to no coating	Scarlet is much deeper red. Coating like this is common for Yin xu.
Pulse: Wiry, rapid	

*This could begin with Liver Yin deficiency leading to Liver Yang rising (as noted), but it could also begin with Kidney Yin deficiency. Per Five Element theory, when the water element (Ki) is deficient in some way, water will fail to feed the wood element of Liver. If that is the case a chart might say something like "Kidney Yin xu causing Liver Yang rising.)

The Lv 3 point on the foot can help root the Liver Yin. Add Ki 3 to this point if there is also Kidney Yin xu.

Here's a mini case study to show you how this might present in clinic:

45 y.o man, chief complaint of throbbing headache for four days. He also has dizziness and vertigo on occasion. His face and eyes look very red. He reports tinnitus and palpitations. He seems very irritable and agitated. He doesn't sleep well and when he does his dreams wake him up and are very anxious in tone. He complains of knee weakness and back aches in the lumbar region. His tongue body is red and a bit thin and the coating is very thin as well, especially in the back 1/3 of the tongue. His pulse is wiry and rapid.

This is a Kidney Yin xu causing Liver Yang rising.

Cold in the Liver meridian
This is an excess condition and is very interior.

	S/sx	Notes
✋	Men: Bearing down sensation in the lower abdomen involving testicles	Cold sinking causing this sensation
	Contracted sensation in the scrotum	
	Pain and discomfort are aggravated by cold, alleviated by warmth	Because this is a true cold condition
	Women: cold pain during the periods	Better with warming
	Tongue: white and slippery coating	
	Pulse: deep, wiry and slow	Deep is interior, wiry says Liver is involved, slow due to cold.

This is also called "stirring of Liver wind in the interior. This is another of the excesses, but is a bit of a special case, so I think it warrants its' own section.

Liver wind has several causes and accompanying presentations..

Root of Lv Wind	Presentation
Extreme heat stirring wind	Extreme heat in the body can breed wind just like heat does in the environment. S/sx are: • High fever • Convulsions of limbs, neck rigidity and opisthotonus (state of a severe hyperextension and spasticity in which an individual's head, neck and spinal column enter into a complete "bridging" or "arching" position backward) • Upward staring eyes (eyes rolled back in head) • Coma • Tongue: red or deep red • Pulse: wiry, rapid, forceful.
Yin xu causing the Wind	Liver yin xu will generate deficient heat, which again swirls upward like a little tornado in the body and you've got wind. S/sx: • Trembling in limbs, especially hands/feet – this is due to dryness and thus a lack of nourishment from Lv to sinews. • Dizziness, tinnitus • Yin xu s/sx: tidal fever, five palm heat, dry mouth and throat, emaciation, irritability • Tongue: red w/cracks, little or no fur • Pulse: thin and rapid.
Blood xu	Lv Blood xu can be an extension of Liver Yin xu or could come from blood loss. S/sx: • Dizziness, tinnitus, pallor, pale nails • Tremulous limbs, hand/feet more, muscle contractions, numbness – blood failing to nourish the tissues • Tongue: pale, thin white coat • Pulse: thin

Damp Heat (Yang Huang) in Liver and Gallbladder

From a biomedical standpoint, this is some form of hepatitis, especially during the acute period of the disease. Look for the three yellows in hepatitis cases – yellow of the sclera, yellow on the skin, bright yellow urine.

Type of Hepatitis	Notes
Hepatitis A	This is acute hepatitis and is passed fecally and orally. There's a vaccine for this. S/sx are: • Abdominal discomfort • Hypochrondria pain • Poor appetite • Nausea • Jaundice • Fatigue
Hepatitis B	Blood borne. The onset is insidious and can go chronic easily. There is a vaccine for this. Mild flu-like s/sx at first, progressing to: • Poor appetite or no appetite • Abdominal and hypochondriac pain • Joint pains • Rash • Chills • Diarrhea These s/sx last 2-6 weeks. Then extreme fatigue and depression for several months. Greater chance of Liver cancer afterwards.
Hepatitis C	Also blood borne, but no vaccine exists for it. Acupuncturists and other health care professionals are at risk for this one. Similar to Hep B in that is also gets chronic easily and also can lead to Liver cancer afterwards. S/sx: • Anorexia/no appetite • Nausea • Vomiting • Jaundice

From a Chinese medical perspective, there are two classifications for jaundice: yin huang and yang huang. It probably won't surprise you at this point to learn the yin huang is associated with damp cold (and a dull color of yellow or "huang") while yang huang is associated with damp heat (and a brighter color of yellow or "huang").

S/sx of Yang Huang or Liver/Gallbladder damp heat are very typical of the biomedical description of hepatitis. This is basically a damp heat pattern which can produce hepatitis symptoms, or shingles (herpes zoster). Look for the 3 yellows: skin, eyes, urine, all bright yellow.

	S/sx	Notes
🖐	Hypochondriac distension and pain	
	Bitter taste in the mouth	Which can be Lv, Gb, or St heat…but is Lv/Gb in this case.
	Nausea/vomiting	
	Abdominal distention	
	Scanty and very yellow urine	
	Yellow sclera	
	Yellow skin on entire body	Also, a very shiny look to the skin.
	Fever	Not usually a high fever due to the dampness.
	Tongue: red body, sticky yellow coating	
	Pulse: rapid, wiry	

Shingles, which is herpes zoster, is damp heat on the surface – red heat circling around the waist or along the nerve channels. The pathway will often, but not always, follow the Gb or Lv channels. Regardless, this is still damp heat in the gallbladder channel.

The acupuncture treatment for this could include Gb 34 and Gb 41. Gb 41 is the exit point of the Gallbladder channel. It opens the door to let the fire disperse. Herbs are also very important for herpes or herpes zoster. Use yin chen hao, and long dan cao, both bitter herbs that clear heat. There is an excellent formula called Long Dan Xie Gan Tang that clears fire from the Liver and Gallbladder.

Disturbance of Phlegm Due to Gallbladder Stagnation

This happens when Gallbladder Qi is not moving and is stagnated. This is very damp related, but the heat from the stagnation cooks the damp down to phlegm. Because the Qi isn't moving, the damp and phlegm aren't either.

It's easy to mistake for this for Heart fire. There is insomnia in the Gallbladder pattern, but no Heart s/sx (like red tongue tip, etc Watch for the *palpitations with fear* to pinpoint this pattern.

That said, unless you treat emotional problems you may never see this. This pattern is not so widely seen.

	S/sx	Notes
	Irritability	
	Insomnia	
✋	Palpitations with fear	Very specific to this pattern.
	Bitter taste in the mouth	
	Nausea and/or vomiting	
	Hypochondriac and chest tightness.	
	Dizziness	
	Tinnitus	

	Tongue: yellow and greasy coating	
	Pulse: wiry and slippery	

There are two fun terms about the Gallbladder in Chinese medicine.

Dan Da	This means "big gallbladder." It means you are very brave and can make decisions quickly and easily.
Dan Xiao	That means "small gallbladder." If the gallbladder is congested you are not brave but fearful.

Dan Xiao is what is happening when the Gallbladder is stagnant and congested. To treat this problem, get rid of damp and phlegm and soothe the Liver. You might use herbs like chai hu to soothe liver and perhaps add ban xia or cang zhu to remove the dampness.

Study Questions

If you haven't made your Liver/Gallbladder Zangfu comparison charts yet, get busy.

Question	Answers
What the key symptom of Liver Qi stagnation?	Distending or wandering pain in the costal and/or hypochondriac regions. Hypochondriac pain is the more common of the two.
How might Liver Qi stagnation lead to Liver wind?	Stagnation leads to heat. Heat generates wind in the body just like it does in the environment.
What are the s/sx of Liver Qi stagnation you could expect to see in a woman of reproductive age? (i.e., older than a kid, younger than menopause)	<ul><li>Breast distention around the periods</li><li>PMS syndrome</li><li>Irregular menstruation</li><li>Lower abdominal cramping, especially before the period starts.</li></ul>
What is the hallmark symptom of Liver Blood xu?	<ul><li>Eye stuff. Specifically:<ul><li>Blurry vision (this is the really big one)</li><li>Dry eyes</li><li>Night blindness</li></ul></li></ul>
How might Liver Blood xu lead to Liver wind?	Blood xu means insufficient volume, which means it stagnates easily. Then stagnation leads to heat, which leads to wind.
How can Liver Blood xu cause dizziness?	<ul><li>Can be Blood xu leading to stagnation, heat, then wind.</li><li>Can be because insufficient blood to nourish the head and brain, then dizziness.</li></ul>
What is the connection between	Nails are considered to be

fingernails and Liver?	continuations of the tendons and sinews, tissues that are controlled by Liver.
What is the key symptom of Liver Yin xu?	Slight burning pain in the hypochondriac area.
How does a Liver Yin xu pulse differ from any other Yin xu?	• Yin xu is thin/thready and rapid. • Liver Yin xu is thin/thready and rapid *and wiry*.
How are Liver Yin xu and Liver Yang rising related?	• Liver Yin xu is the beginning or precursor to Liver Yang rising. • Liver Yin anchors Liver Yang. When this anchor is weak, the Liver Yang can float upward.
Name an emotion that can cause an excess Liver Yang rising. Is this a deficiency or an excess? Is it long term or short term?	• Sudden extreme anger can cause an.... • Excess leading to Liver Yang rising, but this is usually • Short term
What is the deficiency of Liver that can lead to Liver Yang rising?	• Liver Yin xu.
What would a Liver Yang Rising headache look like?	• Distending or throbbing, often at the vertex of the head.
What other organ is likely to be impacted when a patient has Liver dysfunction?	• Kidney. They are besties.
If the Liver has a Yin xu, which other organ will also have a Yin xu?	• Kidney. Kidney Yin xu and Liver Yin xu often come as a "pack."

What type of headache are you likely to see in Liver Fire flaring?	• Distending/throbbing pain, usually at the vertex but could also be at the temples.
Which is considered the more severe condition: Liver Fire Flaring or Liver Yang Rising?	• Liver Yang Rising (I still think this sounds like a bad sci fi novel from the 70's)
Which is more likely to have the sign of hematemesis (vomiting blood) or hemoptysis (coughing/spitting blood)? Liver Fire Flaring or Liver Yang Rising?	• Liver Fire Flaring
What are the s/sx of Liver Wind arising from Liver Yin xu?	• Trembling in the limbs, especially the hands and feet • Dizziness, tinnitus • Yin xu s/sx: tidal fever, five palm heat, night sweats, etc. • Red cracked tongue with little/no coat • Thin rapid pulse
What are the s/sx of Liver Wind coming from Liver Blood xu?	• Liver Blood s/sx: dizziness, tinnitus, pallor, pale nails, etc. • Trembling limbs (esp hands/feet), muscle contractions and numbness.
What are the s/sx of Liver Wind coming from *extreme* heat?	• High fever • Convulsions, neck rigidity, opisthotonus • Upward staring eyes • Coma • Red or deep red tongue body • Wiry, rapid, forceful pulse
What is the hallmark s/sx of cold retention in the Liver meridian?	• Bearing down sensation in the lower abdomen around the genital area (testicles for men).

What is Yang Huang?	• Damp heat in the Liver and Gallblader

While there is no "hallmark" s/sx for Damp Heat in the Liver and Gallbladder, what are you looking for that lets you know exactly what this is?	• Jaundice!
	  o Yellowed sclera - whites of the eyes
	  o Yellow shiny looking skin all over the body
	  o Bright yellow urine

What biomedical diagnosis could Damp Heat in the Gallbladder and Liver be linked to?	• Hepatitis
What Gallbladder related dysfunction looks a lot like Heart fire?	• Disturbance of phlegm due to Gallbladder stagnation
What is the key symptom of disturbance of phlegm due to Gallbladder stagnation?	• Palpitations *with fear*
What other syndrome could have palpitations with fear?	• Trick question. None of them. Only disturbance of phlegm due to Gallbladder stagnation
Why so many heat signs in disturbance of phlegm due to Gallbladder stagnation?	Because stagnation leads to heat and this stagnation has been workin' its' stuff for a while.
OK, what *are* the s/sx of heat in the disturbance of phlegm due to Gallbladder stagnation syndrome?	• Irritability • Insomnia • Bitter taste in the mouth • Yellow tongue coating
How is the tongue coating different between Heart fire and disturbance of phlegm due to Gallbladder stagnation?	• Heart fire: red tongue tip • Disturbance of phlegm due to Gallbladder stagnation: yellow, greasy tongue coating

Now go make your Liver/Gallbladder s/sx charts! Study the hell out of them. **Know the hallmark signs and symptoms.** Know them in your sleep.

This page intentionally left blank
for your non-reading pleasure.

Diagnostics of Chinese Medicine:
Symptom Analysis and Syndrome Differentiation

CHAPTER 10
Kidney and Urinary Bladder

The energy of the Kidney is one of water and fire. The water, Kidney Yin, cools and moistens the body while the fire, Kidney Yang and Mingmen fire, warms and animates. The Yin and Yang of Kidney are the foundation of Yin and Yang in every other organ in the body.

I'll quickly review the Kidney's role in the body to help you understand the pathologies later in this chapter.

Kidney	Brief Discussion
Root of preheaven Qi	The downloaded starter pack from your parents.
Most important organ for men	Liver guides the rhythm of life for women, Kidney for men.

Stores essence	• Governs birth, growth, development
	  If a child isn't developing as she/he should, kidney essence needs work.
	• Governs reproduction
	  o Governs sexual development
	  o Supports pregnancies
	  o Declines during menopause
	• Essence is the material basis for kidney yin/yang

Produces marrow	Fills/strengthens both bone and brain
Controls the reception of Qi	And the breath
Governs water	
Controls the lower 2 orificies	Anus, urethra and spermatic duct.

While the Kidney is related to water and fire, the Bladder is all about water. The relationship between the two of them is an internal/external one. The Bladder needs the fire of the Kidney to transform the water of the body and the Kidney relies on the Bladder to more and excrete waste fluids.

There are many things you will see in clinic that relate to the function of dysfunction of this Yin/Yang pair: UTIs, bladder infections, menopause difficulties, gynecological diseases, enlarged prostate and other genital problems, diabetes*, STDs, congenital disorders, infertility/impotence, sexual dysfunctions, edema, bedwetting, osteoporosis, early morning diarrhea, asthma….. I could go on, but you get the idea.

When discussing the pathologies of the Kidney from a Chinese medical perspective, it is important to know that the Kidneys never have excess. Never. Not once. Don't listen to anyone who tells you differently. Never, never, never, never sedate or reduce the Kidneys!

Kidney has no excess!

The Kidney is the root of the body. No excess.

As a matter of fact, Kidney pathologies are chronic and deficient in nature. Pathologies manifest in one of three basic ways:
- Dysfunction in storing essence
- Disturbance of water metabolism
- Abnormal growth, development, or reproduction

Because Kidney pathologies are more often chronic than acute, alleviation of symptoms will be relatively slow.

There are five Kidney deficiencies to discuss in this chapter. And how many excesses are there? None. Exactly.

Kidney Deficiencies
Kidney Qi xu
Kidney Yang xu
Kidney Yin xu
Kidney Essence xu
Failure of the Kidney to receive Qi

You'll notice here are no tiny hands in the Kidney deficiency lists. Why? Because the whole thing is one giant hand.

Know the Kidney syndromes. Know them so well that you can spot them in the dark without a flashlight. Seriously.

Kidney Qi Xu

Ki Qi Xu s/sx	Brief discussion
Frequent micturition (urination) with clear urine	These are frequent chief complaints – urinary frequency, dribbling.
Dribbling of urine after urination or enuresis	Can afflict men with prostate problems, can occur in people who wet the bed (kids *and* older adults). Expressed in TCM as: "Kidney qi failing to hold firm"
Soreness and weakness of the lumbar region and knee joints	Lower back and knee joints are the Kidney's domain. Problems here can signal Ki xu.
Women: • Clear, cold leucorrhea • Threatened spontaneous abortion	Vaginal discharge is either yellow or white, most of that is mucus. White is cold, yellow is hot. No surprise there. Energy of Kidney is what supports a fetus.
Men: • Spermatorrhea • Premature ejaculation	Spermatorrhea is leakage of sperm. Both of these problems are "Ki Qi failing to hold firm."
Tongue: pale with white coating	Pale shows the cold.
Pulse: deep, weak	Root will also be weak.

Kidney Yang Xu

Yang xu is Qi xu at an advanced stage. You will see more cold s/sx in this set.

Ki Yang xu s/sx	Brief discussion
Pallor or blackish complexion	This is a Five Element association – color is black for Kidney/water
Cold limbs	Common s/sx in Yang xu
Soreness and weakness of lumbar region and knee joints	Same in Ki Qi xu. Why? Because Yang xu and Qi xu share the same root problem.
Impotence	Ki qi is unable to support reproductive function.
Infertility	
Dizziness	Yang Qi cannot ascend to support the head
Cock's crow diarrhea	Diarrhea around 5am-ish, worse when the weather is cold
Edema	
Tongue: pale swollen body, white coat	Water and cold sign
Pulse: deep, weak, probably slow	Deep is interior, weak is xu, slow is cold

You can treat this well with moxibustion. Use a moxa box with a lid, which helps contain the smoke and push it downward toward the body. Place it on the waistline of the back with the center at Du 4, light all of the cones and put the lid on. You could also use warm needle methods at Du 4 and Ren 4. If you treat herbally, there are many excellent formula options such as You Gui Wan. Warm herbs such as rou cong rong and fu zi are often used.

Kidney Yin Xu

We have talked about this a lot. The s/sx should look hella familiar by now. Where Ki Yang xu had many deficient cold s/sx, this dysfunction brings the xu heat.

Ki Yin xu s/sx	Brief discussion
Dizziness, tinnitus	Tinnitus is probably low in volume with a high pitched sound.
Soreness and weakness of lumbar region and knee joints	Kidney xu expresses in lower back and knees
Nocturnal emissions	Men, mostly, but for women leucorrhea could increase at night
Irregular menstruation	Because the Ki is responsible for sexual function and reproductive function
Dry mouth/throat	
Tidal/afternoon fevers	
Malar flush	
Night sweats	....you know...
Darker yellow urine	
Constipation	
Tongue: red with little coating	
Pulse: thin, thready, rapid	

Remember how Kidney Yang xu was treated with an herbal Rx called *You* Gui Wan? Well, Kidney Yin is frequently treated with an herbal prescription called *Zuo* Gui Wan. That's not the only one, but it's one of several. Kidney 3 is the go-to point for Kidney Yin problems.

Kidney Essence Xu

Ki Essence xu s/sx	Brief discussion
Kids: • Delayed growth • Dwarfism • Mental retardation	Essence governs development. Essence xu is unable to do some or all of these things.
Adults: • Sperm defects • Infertility • Amenorrhea • Senilism • Tinnitus, deafness • Poor memory	Improper development of sperm in men Both male and female Failing to supports reproductive function. Premature aging, including premature balding Probably long term
Tongue: red body, white coating	
Pulse: thready, weak	

Acupuncture treatment would include Du 4 and Gb 39 (marrow) points.

Failure of Kidney to Receive Qi

Frequently seen in clinic. This is a big part of asthma – the Lungs inhales, but it is the Kidney that roots the breath, holding it long enough to extract Da Qi (nutrients from breathing). When the Kidney is weak, this doesn't happen efficiently, so there is shortness of breath.

S/sx	Brief discussion
Sore/weak lumbar, knees	
Shortness of breath	Possibly cough too.
Easy exhale, harder inhale	This aggravated by exercise.
Feeble voice	Qi deficiency
Fatigue	
Spontaneous sweating	
Tongue: slightly pale, white coating	
Pulse: deep and weak	

The Bladder is responsible for removing water via Qi transformation. Ki Yang warms the bladder and makes urination easier. Without this warming function, there is retention of urine.

Pathological changes of bladder manifest as abnormal urination such as anuria (lack of micturition, aka urination), urgency of micturition, dysuria, frequency of micturition, incontinence of urine, and enuresis (involuntary night time micturition).

The big one to know for now is damp heat in the Bladder. You'll cover several more Lin syndromes in treatment of disease classes. This particular pathology is the most frequent case of *Lin Zheng* (painful urination).

Western medicine usually assumes this is a bacterial infection and treats with antibiotics, but in Chinese medicine this can be a product of heat, Qi stagnation, and other forms of Lin.

Damp Heat in the Bladder

Note the return of the little hand 🖐. But there's only one of them.

	S/sx	Notes
🖐	Burning pain (heat) in the urethra/during urination	Heat s/sx
	Frequency, urgency of urination	This is heat pushing the urine downward.
	Dribbling of urination	
	Discontinuation of urine in mid-stream	This can be a sign of bladder or urinary stones. This is often painful. The stone blocks the flow or urine causing the discontinuation. Change body position and will often move and urine starts again.

	Dark yellow urine Possible hematuria and/or stones	Heat s/sx
	Lower abdominal distention	Heat and damp in the Bladder.
	Fever	Heat s/sx
	Inflammation	Heat s/sx
	Lumbar pain	Signal that Ki is involved somehow
	Tongue: greasy, yellow coating	Greasy = damp, yellow is heat
	Pulse: rapid	Heat s/sx

To treat this you could use Bladder points, including UB 63, the xi cleft point of the Bladder meridian.

Mini case study:
Two guys walk into a bar…. both have bloody urination. One is young, one is old. The young guy has pain, while the old guy has no pain. Who has the better prognosis?

Young guy. That's probably damp heat. Old guy without pain might have a tumor. Pain is almost always better, strangely enough. Means you are still strong enough to fight.

Study Questions

If you haven't made your Kidney/Bladder Zangfu comparison charts yet, get busy.

Question	Answers
Name a Kidney excess.	Trick question. You can't. There aren't any.
Soreness and weakness in what part of the body is related to Kidney dysfunction?	• Lower back • Knees
What kind of s/sx would you see in women with Kidney Qi xu?	• Clear, cold leuccorhea • Difficulty maintaining a pregnancy.
What kind of s/sx would you see in men with Kidney Qi xu?	• Spermatorrhea • Premature ejaculation
What sign do you see in Kidney Yang xu that you don't see in any other syndrome?	Early morning diarrhea (around 5am, also called cock's crow diarrhea) that is worse in cold weather.
What are the cold s/sx in a Kidney Yang xu?	• Pallor or dark/blackish complexion • Cold limbs • Early morning diarrhea that is worse when it is cold outside • Pulse is deep, weak, **slow**
Kidney Yin xu has Yin xu heat s/sx. That's a given. What are the other s/sx of a Kidney Yin xu?	• Dizziness • Tinnitus (probably high pitched, soft) • Sore, weak lower back and knees • Nocturnal emissions • Irregular menstruation

What kind of s/sx do you see in kids who have a Kidney essence xu?	• Delayed growth and/or closing of the fontanelles • Dwarfism • Mental retardation • And any other genetic defect type problems
How does Kidney Essence xu present in adults?	• Defects of sperm • Male and female infertility • Amenorrhea • Premature balding and other s/sx of Senilism • Tinnitus and deafness • Poor memory (usually long term)
What biomedical disease are you likely to see in someone who has a differentiation of Failure of Kidneys to Receive Qi?	• Asthma
Failure of Kidneys to Receive Qi – list the s/sx.	• Soreness, weakness of lower back and knees • Shortness of breath, maybe cough • Easy to exhale, but difficult to inhale. Worse with exertion. • Feeble voice • Fatigue • Spontaneous sweating • Slightly pale tongue with white coat • Deep, weak pulse
What is the key s/sx of Damp Heat in the Bladder	• Burning pain in the urethra, esp during urination

Do your charts, *know those s/sx and how to tell one of these syndromes from another!* Know your hallmark s/sx

CHAPTER 11
Combination Zangfu Syndromes

Living beings are *complex* physical, emotional, and spiritual entities. Unfortunately for medical students of all varieties, this means that people (or any other animated being) rarely have a single aspect that is out of balance or in a disease state.

That's why we learn combination syndromes. Syndromes usually come in pairs (if you are lucky) or in multiple sets. The older a patient gets the more the combinations multiply.

Here's an example from some old patient files. I've changed a few details, but the basic syndromes expressed are consistent.

A woman has a baby who seems to have chronic digestive problems, possibly because the woman cannot breastfeed and has no access to quality formula. The baby seems healthy despite bouts of colic. The child's caregiver dies when the child is five years old. The child is soon hospitalized with a respiratory disorder and nearly dies, but recovers. The child is diagnosed with asthma and suffers from this for the rest of her life.

As a teen she has chronic recurrent eczema. She also gets colds easily and has seasonal allergies. Her diet is pretty poor with a lot of processed foods and only a few fruits and vegetables. She develops a weight problem and dislikes physical activity as her energy is usually poor.

Later in life her periods become heavy with dark bloods and large clots. This persists into her twenties. In her thirties her partner tells her he cannot take her temper swings or extreme PMS any longer and leaves. This cycle is repeated throughout her 30's and early 40's. Her periods become very light, scanty, and watery in nature. In her 50's she develops calf cramps at night that impair her sleep, and muscle twitches.

Looking back through this woman's history and chart it is clear you could track the path of Spleen Qi deficiency then Lung Qi deficiency (earth unable to generate metal). You can see Liver Qi stagnation developing with heavy blood flow during the periods and then Liver Blood deficiency that persists into her mid adult years. If you treated her in her teens and 20's you would be facing Spleen Qi xu + Liver Qi stagnation + Lung Qi xu.

I didn't take it this far, but in her menopausal history the s/sx of Kidney and Liver yin deficiency were pretty strong. She developed Parkinson's in her late 60's, a Liver wind presentation, quite possibly an offshoot from her chronic Liver Blood xu.

See what I mean? This can get complex. I don't talk about this to freak you out. You will develop treatment strategies to deal with complex cases in the near future. Strategies like focusing on the chief complaint and making sure you are addressing that, using Eight Principles if you get lost in the weeds, and more will get you past the hard parts!

Moving on.

We are going to talk about twelve of the most common combinations you will see in clinic. These are

Heart and Lung Qi xu
Deficiency of Heart and Spleen
Heart and Liver Blood xu
Heart and Kidney Yang xu
Heart and Kidney disharmony

Lung and Spleen Qi xu
Liver fire insulting Lung
Lung and Kidney Yin xu
Liver and Kidney Yin xu
Spleen and Kidney Yang xu
Liver and Spleen disharmony
Liver and Stomach disharmony

All of these can be grouped into a couple of categories: the first five are Heart related. The following three are Lung conditions. The following two are primarily Kidney and the final two are Liver. Looking at it a different way, the top eight are upper jiao, then you see lower jiao and then middle jiao in the final two.

Treatment and study exercise:

Create your own charts for all of the single syndromes and all of the combination syndromes. Do it in your own words. Do it over and over again until you know it well enough that it becomes concise reference.

Not only will this help you learn it, you will create a cool set of cheat sheets for yourself to use in student clinic.

Mine looked like this:

Combination Syndrome	Symptom	Caused by
Qi Deficiency of Heart and Lung	Palpitation	Indicative of heart problem
	Cough with difficult inhalation, worse on exertion	Cough = lung, exert = Qi xu
	Chest tightness	Phlegm ret, Qi congestion,
	Clear phlegm	Dampness MJ, no heat
Upper Jiao problem	Pallor of face	Qi/Yang/Blood Xu or Cold
	Dizziness	Can be excess, or Blood Deficiency
	Lassitude	Qi Xu
	Spontaneous sweating	Qi and Yang Xu
	Tongue: pale with thin white coat	
	Pulse: deep, weak *or* irregular	Deep = interior, weak = deficiency
Deficiency of Heart and Spleen	Palpitations	Heart
	Poor memory	Blood deficiency
Specific pattern in TCM!!!	Insomnia, DDS (dream disturbed sleep)	Heart Qi Xu
This is spleen qi xu + Heart Blood Xu.		Heart of Liver Blood Xu (cant stay asleep, esp elder patients)
Chief complaint often insomnia	Dizziness and vertigo	Can be excess, or Blood Deficiency
	Sallow complexion	Dampness plus Spleen Qi Xu
	Reduced appetite	Spleen
	Abdominal distention	Spleen
	Loose stool, diarrhea	Spleen Qi Xu
	Lassitude	Qi Xu
Middle Jiao problem	Bruising	Spleen Xu, Heat, Trauma
	Scanty and light menses	Blood Xu (thinner and lighter in color) Yin Xu (redder) *If heavy can be blood heat or spleen qi xu*
	Tongue: Pale with white coat	
Gui Pi Tang is the formula of choice	Pulse: Thin and weak	

I used to have them available for download, but many of your instructors e-mailed me to ask that I stop because they felt it was important for students to create their own so that they learned the syndromes better.

There are a few tiny hands in the s/sx lists below to draw your attention and a bold or two here and there. . . but you really just need to know these well enough that you can spot them easily.

HEART AND LUNG QI DEFICIENCY

Heart and Lung Qi xu is definitely an upper jiao problem.

Ht and Lu Qi xu s/sx	Possible indications and notes
Palpitation	• Indicates Heart is affected
Cough with difficult inhalation, worse on exertion	• Coughing indicates Lung. • Worse with exertion points to Qi xu.
Chest tightness	• Retention of phlegm • Qi congestion
Clear phlegm	• Dampness from Middle Jiao Remember that the MJ generates phlegm, the Lu stores it. • Clear tells you no heat involved
Pale face/pallor	• Qi xu • Yang xu • Blood xu • Cold
Dizziness	• Possible excess cause • Blood xu
Lassitude	• Qi xu
Spontaneous sweating	• Qi xu • Yang xu
Tongue: pale with thin white coat	
Pulse: either deep and weak *or* irregular	Deep/weak = interior xu

Points you could use for this would include (but are not limited to) Ht 7 and Lu 9 on the upper extremities, as well as Bl 15 (back shu of the Heart) and Bl 13 (back shu of the Lung).

Diagnostics of Chinese Medicine:
Symptom Analysis and Syndrome Differentiation

This is a *very specific combination in clinic*. It is actually a Spleen Qi xu combined with Heart Blood xu. Do not confuse it with anything else Heart and Spleen related!

The patient's chief complaint is often insomnia. This is considered to be a middle jiao problem, but you can see both the middle and upper jiao's affected here.

Xu of Ht and Sp s/sx	Possible indications and notes
Palpitations	• Tells you the Heart is involved
Poor memory	• Blood xu • Can also implicate Ht or Ki
Insomnia with DDS	DDS is "dream disturbed sleep." You'll probably see this in charts. • Heart Qi xu • Heart Blood xu • Liver Blood xu Heart related insomnia is generally trouble getting to sleep. Liver is often trouble *staying* asleep, waking around 2-4 am.
Dizziness and vertigo	• Can be due to excess causes • Can be due to Blood xu
Sallow complexion	• Dampness + Spleen Qi xu
Reduced appetite	• Spleen is affected
Abdominal distention	
Loose stool, diarrhea	• Spleen Qi xu
Lassitude	• General Qi xu

Easy bruising	• Spleen Qi xu
	   Skin bruises very easily – sign that the Spleen is unable to hold blood
	• Heat in the Blood
	   This can cause reckless bleeding – blood moves faster with heat and can punch through the bonds that hold the single layer of epithelial cells that make up the capillaries. That lets the blood leak out of the capillaries and causes the bruising.
	• Trauma can also cause bruising, but that's kind of a different story.

Scanty and light menses	• Blood xu Blood will be thinner and lighter in color. May have a "watercolor" look to it. • Yin xu Blood will be redder in color than with Blood xu Heavy bleeding can indicate Blood heat or Spleen Qi xu.
Tongue: Pale body, white coat	
Pulse: Thin and weak	

Gui Pi Tang is the herbal formula of choice for this combination syndrome. Points you might choose for this could include: Ht 7, St 36, Sp 6, Li 10 (to boost Wei qi), Bl 17 and Bl 15. You would choose tonification methods and points.

HEART AND LIVER BLOOD XU

This lower jiao combination is seen rather often in anemia patients. You can also see this condition in psoriasis patients. This is the chronic phase of psoriasis, not the acute type which is characterized by itching.

Look for the very specific symptom of tremors below.

Ht and Lv Blood Xu	Possible indications and notes
Palpitations	• Tells you the Heart is involved
Poor memory	• Blood xu • Can also implicate Ht or Ki
Insomnia with DDS	DDS is "dream disturbed sleep." You'll probably see this in charts. • Heart Qi xu • Heart Blood xu • Liver Blood xu Heart related insomnia is generally trouble getting to sleep. Liver is often trouble *staying* asleep, waking around 2-4 am.
Dizziness and vertigo	• Can be due to excess causes • Can be due to Blood xu
Pale face	• Qi xu

	• Yang xu • Blood xu • Cold
Dry eyes	• Lv Yin xu (also Blood xu)
Blurred vision	This isn't "I need glasses" blurry, but uncorrectable kind of blurry. • Lv Yin xu advancing or advanced to Lv Blood xu
Numb limbs	Can be due to anemia and malnutrition. Qi and Blood xu can cause this. • Blood xu
🖐 Tremors 🖐	This is a very specific manifestation of this combination syndrome. • Liver Wind • Other s/sx of Lv wind are itching and rashes.
Scanty menses	• Blood xu • Yin xu (with other supporting Yin xu s/sx)
Tongue: Pale body, white coat	
Pulse: Thin, weak	

HEART AND KIDNEY YANG XU

This is a bit of a tricky pattern. Don't confuse it with a Heart Kidney disharmony, which is a really specific Yin xu combination syndrome and diagnosis pattern. (See the next syndrome for Heart Kidney disharmony.) That helps you tell the difference between Heart and Kidney Yang xu and Heart Kidney disharmony.

Many chronic heart failure patients have this combination syndrome. They often want to cover their chest because it feels sensitive to cold.

Ht and Ki Yang Xu	Possible indications and notes
Palpitations	• Tells you the Heart is involved
Pale face	• Qi xu • Yang xu • Blood xu • Cold
Aversion to cold, cold limbs	• Yang xu • Also extreme anger causing Qi congestion
Sleepy often	• Heart Qi xu – the most likely suspect • Spleen Qi xu – more likely after meals because energy is diverted to digestion after eating…and there's not much to spare!
Edema in face and limbs, especially in the lower legs	• Kidney Yang xu when edema is in lower limbs. Water cannot be steamed away because there is insufficient fire, so gathers and gets swampy in the lower limbs. • Spleen xu – this is edema in *all four* limbs. • Qi stagnation – this is non-pitting edema.
Cold, soreness, and weakness in the lumbar area and in the knee joints	• Kidney Yang xu with deficient cold
Pale lips and nails	• Blood xu • Qi xu • Yang xu
Early morning diarrhea	Diarrhea around 5am-ish, diarrhea problem gets more severe when the weather is cold. • Kidney Yang xu – really typical s/sx
Tongue: Pale body, slippery coat	Could be either of these, but both will have water retention. (Slippery coat) • Yang xu • Qi xu
Pulse: Deep, feeble, slow	• Deep shows interior/longterm problem • Feeble shows xu • Slow slows the cold

As with any of the Yang xu patients, you could use moxibustion or warm needling. Du 4 would be a great place for that. Use acupuncture at Ht 7.

HEART AND KIDNEY DISHARMONY

There are two basic relationships between Heart and Kidney: Heart and Kidney Yang xu and Heart and Kidney Yin xu. This second one, deficiency of both Heart and Kidney is so common it has the special syndrome name of Heart and Kidney disharmony.

There is a unique relationship between Heart and Kidney– the relationship of fire and water. These must be balanced or the water will overpower and extinguish the fire…or the fire will boil the water away. If water is too little, cannot nourish the heart, the fire gets too strong and burns the kidney, burns away more water.

Here are the signs and symptoms for a Heart Kidney disharmony.

Ht Ki disharmony s/sx	Possible indications and notes
Palpitations	• Tells you the Heart is involved
Insomnia	• Heart Qi xu • Heart Blood xu • Liver Blood xu Heart related insomnia is generally trouble getting to sleep. Liver is often trouble *staying* asleep, waking around 2-4 am.
Restlessness, irritability	• Heart fire • Liver fire
Poor memory	• Heart Yin xu • Blood xu • Can also implicate Ht or Ki
Dizziness and vertigo	SO many possibilities here. In this case it's probably yin xu in the lower jiao allowing the yang to float upwards.
Tinnitus	• Kidney yin xu
Dry throat	• Yin xu

	(Kidney channel goes to the back of the throat)
Tidal fever	• Yin xu
Night sweating	•
Soreness of lumbar and waist	• Kidney involvement
Spermatorrhea in dreams	• Kidney xu
Tongue: Red body, little to no coating	• Yin xu heat
Pulse: Thin and rapid	• Xu heat

LUNG AND SPLEEN QI DEFICIENCY

Lu and Sp Qi xu	Possible indications and notes
Chronic, constant cough with profuse clear phlegm	• Cough – lung • Phlegm – spleen • Chronic – deficiency • Clear – shows no heat
Shortness of breath	• Lung xu
Poor appetite	• Spleen symptom
Abdominal distention	• Shows Spleen involvement
Loose stools, diarrhea	• Spleen Qi xu

LIVER FIRE INSULTING LUNG

Emotional symptoms usually occur first, followed by fire and heat s/sx.

Lv fire insulting Lu	Possible indications and notes
Burning pain or distension in the hypochondriac or costal areas	The hypochondriac area is also called "flank" in some texts. • Liver indicated Because of the location of the sensations.
Quick temper, irritability	The two primary suspects are these. Probably both in this case • Liver • Heat

Diagnostics of Chinese Medicine:
Symptom Analysis and Syndrome Differentiation

Restlessness	If this sounds like a Heart symptom, you're right. Liver fire (wood element) long term affects the child element of fire or Heart. This is a mother/son relationship.
Dizziness	Again, lots of reasons for dizziness. In this case… • Wind due to excessive heat
Red eyes	Refers to the sclera of the eyes. • Liver fire affecting the eyes
Bitter taste in the mouth	• Liver fire • Stomach fire • Gallbladder fire
Very strong, intermittent cough	Like, this cough is *violent* in nature. That's always an excess. • Shows Lung excess
Sticky scanty yellow phlegm, coughing blood	Also called "spitting blood." • Sticky, little, yellow = heat • Spitting blood = heat • Cough = Lung involvement. This is Liver insulting Lung s/sx.
Hot sensation in the chest	Heat symptom
Tongue: Red body, thin yellow coat	Heat, heat, heat
Pulse: Wiry, rapid	• Wiry = Liver involvement • Rapid = heat

LUNG AND KIDNEY YIN XU

Lu and Ki Yin xu s/sx	Possible indications and notes
Cough plus little sputum or bloody sputum	• Cough indicates Lung involvement • Little points to deficiency • Bloody sputum tells you there heat
Dry mouth and/or sore, dry throat	• Dry points to Yin or Body Fluid xu • Sore throat indicates Lu and Ki channels
Hoarse voice	• Lu yin xu
Losing weight or emaciated	• Yin xu sign

Soreness/weakness of lumbar and knee joints	• Area of the Kidney
Tidal fever	• Yin xu
Malar flush	
Night sweats	
Nocturnal emissions	• Kidney Yin xu
Less menses than previously	• Yin xu
Tongue: Red body, little/no coat	• Red – heat • Little/no coat - xu
Pulse: Thin, rapid	• Thin – xu • Rapid – heat

Patients might also complain of a high-pitched tinnitus. This is a Kidney Yin xu symptom.

LIVER AND KIDNEY YIN XU

This one is fairly common in an aging population. Women in menopause have these s/sx often. As with any syndrome, you probably won't see all of these signs and symptoms, but you'll see enough to spot the syndrome.

Also, don't let the Heart looking s/sx throw you off. This looks a bit like a Heart and Kidney disharmony, but it's not. Heart/Kidney is a fire and water relationship. Liver/Kidney Yin xu is a relationship between Blood and Shen. There are no palpitations here to implicate the Heart, but you do see dry eyes and hypochondriac pain that point to Liver involvement.

Lv and Ki Yin xu s/sx	Possible indications and notes

Dizziness, vertigo	• Interior wind
	Many possible causes for wind
	  ○ Blood xu
	  ○ Excess heat
	  ○ Yin xu w/ xu heat

Tinnitus Probably high pitched	• Kidney yin xu Kidney channel goes to the ears, Kidneys are related to ears also.
Dull hypochondriac	• Dull: deficiency

pain	• Hypochondriac area: Liver/Gallbladder
Poor memory	• Poor short term memory is Ht Blood xu • Poor long term memory is Ki xu
Insomnia with DDS	Several possible causes. Pay attention to *when* the patient has difficult sleeping: • Heart Qi xu • Heart Blood xu • Liver Blood xu Heart related insomnia is generally trouble getting to sleep. Liver is often trouble *staying* asleep, waking around 2-4 am.
Dry throat, mouth, eye	• Liver – Liver opens to the eyes, a part of the meridian goes to the throat. • Dry mouth – yin xu with xu heat damaging fluids.
Losing weight, emaciated	• Yin xu
Soreness/weakness of lumbar and knee joints	• Area of the Kidney
Tidal fever	• Yin xu
Malar flush	
Night sweats	
Nocturnal emissions	• Kidney Yin xu
Less menses than previously	• Yin xu
Tongue: Red body, little/no coat	• Red – heat • Little/no coat - xu
Pulse: Thin, rapid	• Thin – xu • Rapid – heat

Generally best treated with herbs, but you can also use tonification points for Liver and Kidney such as Lv 3 and Ki 3.

SPLEEN AND KIDNEY YANG XU

Sp and Ki Yang xu s/sx	Possible indications and notes
Pale face/pallor	• Yang xu • Qi xu • Blood xu

	• Cold
Poor appetite	• Spleen qi xu
Aversion to cold, cold limbs	• Yang xu Because it is all four limbs, likely Spleen
Cold, soreness and weakness of lumbar and knee joints	• Sore weak lumbar and knee points to Kidney xu • Cold sensation points to Yang xu
Loose stools or diarrhea at dawn; chronic diarrhea	• Early morning diarrhea is Ki Yang xu • Chronic is deficiency
Urinary incontinence	• Ki qi xu • Ki yang xu
Facial puffiness and edema in the limbs	• Edema in the limbs o Can suggest Spleen because it is all four limbs o Can also suggest Sp *and* Ki because edema in the upper body is Sp related, edema below the waist is Ki related. o Facial edema would suggest Sp or Lung, but if it was Lung there would be more of those s/sx.
Tongue: Pale swollen body, slippery white coat	• Pale swollen suggests cold and damp retention here. Slippery coat also points to damp • Pale could also suggest cold.
Pulse: Deep, feeble, slow	• Deep is an interior problem • Feeble is deficiency • Slow is cold

Treat with moxibustion (aka "moxa"). Good points would be Sp 6, Sp 9, and Du 4. A moxa box at Du 4 area would probably feel amazing to this patient.

DISHARMONY OF LIVER AND SPLEEN, DISHARMONY OF LIVER AND STOMACH

Group these two combination syndromes together. This is Liver overacting on the Middle Jiao, or wood over-controlling earth. You might also see this in Chinese medicine charts noted as "Liver overacting on Spleen" or "Liver overacting on Stomach" or even "Liver overacting on Middle Jiao" (when both Sp/St are affected).

Disharmony of Liver and Spleen

Disharmony of Lv/Sp s/sx	Possible indications and notes
Distention/fullness and pain in the hypochondriac or costal area	• This location indicates the Liver is involved
Intermittent sighing for no evident reason	• Liver Qi stagnation
Poor appetite	• Spleen qi xu
Abdominal distention	•
Depression and irritability	• Liver involvement. Depression is often Qi stagnation while irritability is fire
Loose stools or constipation	• Spleen qi xu Could be one or the other. Loose because the Qi can't hold the stool long enough to process or constipation because there isn't enough Qi to push the stool through. Different expression, but the same problem.
Tongue: White and/or greasy coating	• Greasy would be phlegm/damp retention. White could be normal.
Pulse: Wiry	• Points to the Liver.

Disharmony of Liver and Stomach

Liver overacting on the stomach can be due to heat or cold.

- Heat: Liver Qi stagnation can transform to fire which then affects the Stomach
- Cold: retention of cold in the body can affect the balance between the Liver and Stomach

Disharmony of Lv/St s/sx	Possible indications and notes
Distention/fullness and pain in the hypochondriac or costal area	• This location indicates the Liver is involved
Belching, hiccupping, acid reflux	• Liver overacting on Stomach will impair the Stomach's ability to descend Qi, causing the Qi to rebel upward. Patient could also have constipation for this reason.
Irritability	• Heat symptom
Tongue: Red body, thin yellow coat	• Red is heat • And so is yellow
Pulse: Wiry, rapid	• Wiry – Liver • Rapid - heat

Dissect each of these cases and decide which of the syndromes you have studied so far apply. Case study analysis follows the cases.

Case Studies

Case 1: Wanda, 42 year old female, cough for 10 days

Has a cough for 10 days with little sputum that is sticky and yellow. It was severe at the beginning, but alleviated now after taking meds. Currently it is a constant, strong cough and her voice is disturbed. She coughs a lot in the morning, but it's better in the daytime. She mentioned that she had a bad argument with her family 2 weeks ago. Afterwards, she started having headaches in the vertex area, irritability, red and swollen sensation in her eyes, bitter sensation in her mouth, stuffiness in her chest, burning pain in hypochondriac area occasionally. Overall, she feels hot.
Physical assessment: Comprehensive heavy sensation in the chest, heavy breath. Tongue is red in the front and sides of body with thin yellow coating. Pulse is wiry and rapid.

Case 2: Robert, 46 y.o. male, palpitations x4 years, poor appetite for 6 months

Felt the palpitation sensation for 4 years. He's got poor memory and bad concentration. Sometimes it is very difficult for him to focus on his work. He has been to a doc, but no positive or obvious findings to the tests. He doesn't have a good appetite and suffers from gas and bloating after meals. Occasionally he has diarrhea and easily gets bruised. He sleeps badly even when he's exhausted. Has dream disturbed sleep and wakes up tired.
Physical assessment: Pale complexion, soft muscles, no positive physiological reactions, but tends to react slowly. Tongue is pale and swollen with teeth marks, white coat. Pulse is thin and weak.

Case 3: Barry, 70 y.o. male, heart palpitations and diarrhea for 10 years

Palpitations for 10 years. He has been to doc and got EKGs, but everything looks "normal" even with 24 hour monitoring. He feels confused, but didn't know what to do about the situation. He heard about acupuncture and decided to give it a try. He as spontaneous sweating. Sometimes he feels tired and it gets worse with exertion. Appetite is good. He jogs regularly. He usually has a bowel movement early in the morning which varies from loose to watery in nature. He mentioned that he felt cold in the chest and lower back. His urine is clear and usually copious in amount. Occasionally he dribbles (no, not basketball) due to his enlarged prostate. He mentioned he has edema in both lower legs.

Physical assessment: BP is 140/75. Pulse is 76bpm, breath rate is normal.

Tongue: purplish, slippery white coat

Pulse: feeble, slow, deep

Case 4: Austin, 55 y.o. male, fatigue for 3 years

He was very energetic and did mountain bike training for a while. He trained very hard 3 years ago for a national competition. After training very hard he began to feel weak. He tried to remedy this with good rests, sleeping, good foods, but to no positive result. His appetite is poor and he feels tired after he eats. He also notices he feels very full in the epigastrium after eating, even if he eats little meals. His bowels are loose, but no diarrhea. He also coughs sometimes, but it's not bad. He only coughs when he feels weak. The cough produces a profuse amount of sputum. His voice is low and he is short of breath.

Physical assessment: Tongue: pale with teethmarks and a thin white coat. Pulse: weak.

Case Study Analysis

Let's see how well you did. This is a really quick analysis. You could look back through the material and find other possibilities, but look at how the symptoms are stacking up as you read through the case material. Make sure your best guess is supported by the evidence.

Case 1: Wanda, 42 year old female, cough for 10 days

S/sx	Possible indications and notes
Cough	Lung
Little sputum, sticky, yellow	Heat, and it's affecting Body Fluids and Lung moisture.
Severe cough both at onset and current	Lung excess
Coughing in the morning	Lung Qi is disturbed by her change of physical position when she gets up out of bed

Quarreled with her family 2 weeks ago	• Emotional turmoil leading to fire in liver.
	   o Afterwards got the vertex headache, irritability, red/swollen eyes, bitter sensation in the mouth, burning pain in the hypochondriac area = Liver fire
	   o Also note that she mentioned chest stuffiness in this litany… fire going up to the Lung.

General hot feeling	• Heat
Comprehensive heavy sensation in the chest	• Lung area • Also could be phlegm or Qi stagnation causing the heaviness
Breathing hard	• Lung excess
Tongue: Red body front and sides with thin yellow coat	• Red in front = Ht or Lu heat • Red on sides = Lv or Gb heat • Coat is heat
Pulse: Wiry, rapid	• Wiry = Liver • Rapid = heat

What is this? Liver fire insulting Lung

Case 2: Robert, 46 y.o. male, palpitations x4 years, poor appetite for 6 months

S/sx	Possible indications and notes
Palpitations for 4 years	• Chronic situation • Heart involvement
Poor appetite for ½ year	• Spleen qi xu
Poor memory, bad concentration Difficult to focus	• Heart Blood xu
Went to the doc and no conclusive results	• Ugh! So frustrating
Doesn't have a good appetite Easily bruised	• Spleen Qi xu • Bruising is Spleen unable to hold Blood in vessels in this case
Sleeps badly	• Heart Blood xu?
Vivid-dreaming during sleep	• Heart Blood disturbed by either heat or xu
Wakes tired	• Spleen Qi xu

What is going on with Robert? Deficiency of Heart and Spleen

Case 3: Barry, 70 y.o. male, heart palpitations and diarrhea for 10 years

S/sx	Possible indications and notes
Palpitations	• Heart involvement
Diarrhea for 10 years	• Spleen or Kidney • Chronic problem, regardless of organ involved.
Appetite is fine	• Ok, so maybe not Spleen involvement. (Could also be that this s/sx just isn't showing up yet. Or Barry uses a decent amount of cannabis. I'm not being facetious. Stuff shows up in clinic like this – lifestyle habits mitigating or changing s/sx you'd expect to see.)
Spontaneous sweating	• Qi xu • Yang xu
Tired feeling, worse w/ exertion	• Qi xu
Early a.m. bowels - loose to watery	• Ki Yang xu
Cold in the chest	• Heart or Lung – could be excess or xu • Yang xu
Cold in the lower back	• Kidney area, Yang xu
Urine is clear, copious	• Could be excess interior cold or deficiency cold… • But clear and profuse is *so* Yang xu
Dribbling of urine	• Kidney xu
Edema, both legs	• Kidney yang xu, not enough heat to transform and steam the moisture up, so it's building up in the lower limbs.
Tongue: Purple body, slippery white coat	• Purple is stasis • Slippery white coat is damp or water retention, no heat
Pulse: Deep, feeble, slow	• Deep is interior and/or chronic • Feeble is deficiency • Slow is cold

What does this add up to? Yang xu of Heart and Kidney

Case 4: Austin, 55 y.o. male, fatigue for 3 years

S/sx	Possible indications and notes
Fatigue	• Qi xu, likely to be Sp
Tired after training very hard	• The dude burned away some Qi! All things in moderation, Crossfit Grasshopper! Too much of anything is not great for you.
Weakness after training	• Qi xu
Poor appetite and tired after meals	• Sp qi xu
Epigastric fullness after any meal	• Spleen xu
Bowel is loose, not diarrhea though	• Spleen xu
Coughs, though not bad, when he feels very weak	• Lu xu
Cough with profuse sputum	• Phlegm retention. Middle jiao generates phlegm, but Lung stores it • No heat indicated or the sputum would be yellow, less, sticky.
Low voice, shortness of breath	• Lu qi xu
Tongue: Pale body with teeth marks, thin white coat	• Pale with TM (teeth marks) – Qi xu (probably Sp) with water retention • May be normal, does show there's no heat.
Pulse: Weak	• Xu

What's up with this guy? Spleen and Lung Qi Xu

Make Those Charts!

Have I mentioned you need to do those charts? Because you do. And you need to know that stuff cold. Know the hallmark s/sx!

SECTION 3
Six Channel Theory

This is one of the many ways to categorize and analyze disease progression and helps to determine treatment. Do not rely on any one theory exclusively, but use your intuition along with all of the tools in your toolbox (Eight Principles, Zang Fu Theory, Four Levels, San Jiao Theory, etc.).

This particular theory was developed by Zhang Zhongjing and is detailed in the *Shang Han Lun*. Zhang Zhongjing, regarded as a saint in Chinese medicine, was born in the era of the Han dynasty into a very large family. He became governor of his province in a time when there were many wars and result plagues. During his reign one of these plagues killed a large portion of his family. Thereafter he dedicated his life to studying disease and treatment.

He wrote Shang Han Za Bing Lun, broken into Shang Han Lun (Cold Damage Disease) and Jin Kui Yao Lue (Golden Chamber or cabinet – miscellaneous disease) later. Shang Han Za Bing Lun is related to Cold damage or disease and miscellaneous disease. But because of the turmoil of the region, the book was lost, then recovered in parts and rewritten.

The theory defines stages of diseases in order to determine proper treatment for the patient at each stage. Each is described as a syndrome with specific methods of treatment. Please note that a disease may not play "nice" and go in the order below. Often a disease involves two channels at one time and/or skips a stage all together. Sometimes interior and exterior are mixed, involving both the channel and the organ. Be flexible in your thinking and remember bodies are dynamic things. Rarely will you encounter a textbook *anything*.

Finally, bear in mind that this is a summarized discussion of this theory. For a more complete discussion, refer to a good translation of the *Shang Han Lun.*

The listed order in which disease progresses according to Six Channel Theory:

Taiyang ☞ Yangming ☞ Shaoyang ☞ Taiyin ☞ Shaoyin ☞ Jueyin

You will get a lot more of this in your study of classical disease theories. Three of the progression levels have sub-syndromes to know.

Level	Sub-level
Taiyang Syndrome	Taiyang Zhong Feng Syndrome
	Taiyang Shang Han Syndrome
Yangming Syndrome	Yangming Jing Syndrome
	Yangming Fu Syndrome
Shaoyang Syndrome	
Taiyin Syndrome	
Shaoyin Syndrome	Shaoyin Cold Syndrome
	Shaoyin Heat Syndrome
Jueyin Syndrome	

These relate to Zangfu theory. Please note the chain starts with yang – a more exterior force. The chain ends with Yin, which is deeper and colder.

WHY ARE WE STUDYING THIS?

It's easy to get lost in the weeds when you're cramming data into your brain, so I thought I would mention this.

You're studying this because
1) It's tried and true. This has been proven over a couple thousand years, so it's solid in principle and helps you get patients healthy.

2) The awesome treatment strategies!
   We're not diving into this here, but the herbal treatments coupled with the levels and sublevels you will merely touch on here are mind boggling in their coolness.

   As disease pathogens become more and more resistant to antibiotic overuse and treatments, these studies become even more important. Though the recent swine and avian flu epidemics did not hit North America very hard, they did a lot of damage in Asia and in the eastern hemisphere. Chinese physicians used herbal medicine based on the principles found in the Shang Han Lun (the source for our knowledge of the Six Stages) and Wen Bing (the source for what we know about warm injured disease) to successfully treat these epidemics.

Left it blank on purpose, folks. Yes, I did.

CHAPTER 12
The Exterior Syndromes

The first two stages of the Six Channels Theory of a cold-invading disease are very yang and exterior in nature. The first stage is Taiyang and the second is Yangming. Please note once again, that invading pathogens do not read books. They do whatever they want. *Learn* the stages in order, but don't expect the pathogens to play that nicely all the time.

THE TAIYANG STAGE

Taiyang is the exterior and first stage of disease progression per Six Channel Theory. The disease is just beginning to attack the patient. You'll see chills and fever according to the Eight Principles theory and you see that here too. Patients sometimes feel this on their back as a cold sensation – this is where the Taiyang meridians (Bladder and Small Intestine) runs – up the back, across the upper back and onto the back of the neck. This is where many exterior invasions are felt.

Note that this stage primarily considered to an *attack on the Lung*. Do you see that in the s/sx? No. Not really. But the Lung is the first line of defense in the body and is the most exterior Zang organ you own and since this whole theory is about disease progression, Lung it is.

Taiyang Zhong Feng Syndrome

This is a wind attack version of the Taiyang Syndrome. This is similar to an exterior deficiency or wind heat invasion. The symptoms are below in the table. Note the use of the "pointing finger ☞. This points to the difference between this version of the syndrome and the next one, the Taiyang Shang Han Syndrome.

Mild fever, chills

Aversion to wind

☞ Easily and frequently perspires

Headache

Tongue: Pale body, thin white coating

Pulse: Floating, slowed down

Taiyang Shang Han Syndrome

This looks like an exterior wind cold attack, yes? (Yes. The answer is yes.)

More chills than fever

☞ No sweating!

Headache

Neck and body pain

Tongue: Pale body, thin white coating

Pulse: Floating, slowed down

YANGMING SYNDROMES

This is the second or third stage of a disease's progress… It was the second stage as it was taught to me, but some schools of thought in Chinese medicine put the Shaoyang stage before the Yangming, but traditionally Shaoyang is the "between" stage – sitting between exterior and interior.

Regardless, this is a very important stage in the disease progression because of the richness of the Yangming meridian, which is rich in Qi and Blood resources. Once the disease reaches this stage it has access to great resources, giving it the nutrients to arm itself for further progression into the interior and also access to distribute itself through the Qi and Blood pathways.

This stage is considered to be an attack on the Large Intestine or Stomach. In this case, you really do see s/sx of Large Intestine and Stomach involvement. Note the copious heat signs in this stage of disease. The Yangming channels are the Large Intestine and Stomach channels. They are used often to clear heat.

There are 2 subcategory syndromes of the Yangming stage of disease: Jing or Channel Syndrome and Fu or Organ Syndrome

Yangming Jing Syndrome

You see the Four Greats here – great fever, profuse sweating, great thirst, and a big pulse. Again, I'm using the pointing finger to indicate the differences between the two versions of the Yangming syndrome.

No aversion to cold
☞ No constipation
Red face
High fever
Profuse sweating
Big thirst
Tongue: Red body, yellow dry coating
Pulse: Rapid

You could use Lung 10 and Ren 17 to help with the cough and high fever. Add Li 11 anytime you see heat, as it helps the body to clear any kind.

Yangming Fu or Organ Syndrome

Constant fever, more pronounced in the afternoon
☞ Constipation
Abdominal pain and distention
Tongue: Red body w/prickles, dry thick yellow coat
Pulse: deep, excessive.
Big thirst
Tongue: Red body, yellow dry coating
Pulse: Rapid

You could use LI 11 and Li 2 for heat, Sj 6 and St 37 to help with constipation.

Left this blank on purpose. Yes, I did.

Diagnostics of Chinese Medicine:
Symptom Analysis and Syndrome Differentiation

CHAPTER 13
Shaoyang Syndrome

This is usually considered to be the step between Taiyang and Yangming, and indicates disease progression from exterior to interior (or, if things are improving for this patient, from interior to exterior)– and thus is generally placed between Yangming and Taiyin stages.

It has no subcategories, unlike it's other Yang sisters. The Shaoyang Syndrome corresponds in Zangfu Theory to the Gallbladder and San Jiao. The Yangwei channel is also closely tied to Shaoyang.

A Shaoyang syndrome has a very specific characteristic in that it is half interior, half exterior. Invading pathogens are very close to having access to all of the body's internal resources when a pathogen progresses this far. Look for the fluctuations between the two extremes of expression. I'm once again using the pointing finger ☞ to emphasize the key symptom here.

> ☞ **Alternating chills and fever**
> Bitter taste in the mouth
> Dry throat
> Dizziness and blurred vision
> Poor appetite with nausea and vomiting
> Pain in the hypochondriac region
> Restlessness and irritability
> Tongue: Red sides, either thin white or thin yellow coating, often mixed
> Pulse: Wiry

Bitter taste in the mouth, restlessness and irritability, and the tongue indicates heat, while dry throat is probably because the body is burning off the body fluids with all that heat. You can see the Middle Jiao is affected (n/v) and you also know the Liver is involved by the flank pain and eye s/sx.

Diagnostics of Chinese Medicine:
Symptom Analysis and Syndrome Differentiation

CHAPTER 14
The Interior Syndromes

Once the "line" between exterior and interior has been crossed, the pathogen is firmly in the door. There are three stages indicating progression of a pathogen on the interior of the body: Taiyin, Shaoyin, and Jueyin. Taiyin is the most exterior of the three and Jueyin is the most interior. If a pathogen is allowed to progress from the exterior all the way to the Jueyin stage, the patient will likely die. If a s/sx indicate a pathogen is moving from interior to exterior, then the prognosis is good.

TAIYIN SYNDROME

This is the first level that is considered to be interior. Taiyin Syndrome is also called is also called Greater Yin Syndrome. There are no sub-levels in this syndrome.

The Taiyin Syndrome is predominantly related to the Spleen. If you look at it from a Zangfu perspective, you see that pretty clearly in the signs and symptoms.

> Abdominal fullness and pain
> Nausea/vomiting
> Diarrhea
> Zero thirst
> Tongue: Pale body with a white greasy coating
> Pulse: Deep, slow, weak

These symptoms are characteristic of Spleen Qi xu and the treatment is the same: tonify Spleen using St 36 with moxa and Sp 6. Add Ren 12 for nausea and vomiting and St 25 for diarrhea.

The Shaoyin stage is divided into two sub-syndromes: Shaoyin Cold and Shaoyin Heat. The organs most heavily affected the Kidney and the Heart at this stage of progression and you can see that in the s/sx below.

Shaoyin Cold Syndrome

Looks quite a lot like Kidney Yang deficiency until you get to the pulse, which has a more severe presentation than Ki Yang xu. Cold s/sx here are more severe than you saw in the Taiyin Syndrome and are more focused on the lower areas.

No fever
Aversion to cold with cold limbs
Tendency to sleep a lot, listlessness
Diarrhea with undigested food
Clear urine with increased volume
Tongue: Pale body with white coating
Pulse: Deep, minute

Treat with moxibustion at Du 4 and Ren 4.

Shaoyin Heat Syndrome

Compare this with the Heart/Kidney disharmony .

Restlessness, irritability
Insomnia
Dry mouth and throat
Scanty, deep yellow urination
Tongue: Red body with red tip, very little to no coating
Pulse: Thin, rapid

Tonify the Heart and Kidney Yin with the following points: Kid 3, UB 23, UB 43

JUEYIN SYNDROME

This is also called Terminal Yin Syndrome. . . because if a patient progresses this far, they are likely to be terminal. Because of it's placement in the progression, it's actually a lot more complicated and severe than this makes it sound. If you read the classics, you'll see the possible signs and symptoms are far greater than this short-I'm-just-learning-Chinese-medicine list.

This stage correlates to the Liver and Pericardium.

Heat in the upper, cold in the lower
Thirst
Ascending of Qi to the chest
Burning sensation in the chest
Hungry, but no desire to eat
Vomiting after meals
Tongue: red or pale body
Pulse possibilities: Slippery, deep, weak, hidden

So many organs could be involved that this will cause variations in how the tongue and pulse present, so I'm not even going there with you. More on that in Classics.

Study Questions

Question	Answers
Who developed the Six Channel Theory?	Zhang Zhongjing
What aspect of disease is the Six Channel Theory tracking?	Progression of disease from exterior to interior.
What is the order of a disease's progress per the Six Channel Theory? *(just the main ones, not the subs)*	Taiyang → Yangming → Shaoyang → Taiyin → Shaoyin → Jueyin
What is the Taiyang Zong Feng syndrome similar to from what you have studied previously?	External wind heat invasion
What is the key s/sx of the Taiyang Zong Feng stage that sets it apart from the Taiyang Shang Han version of the Taiyang stage?	Easy sweating, perspires frequently
What is the hallmark s/sx of the Taiyang Shang Han syndrome?	No sweating. None. Zip.
Which of the six stages are considered to be exterior syndromes?	Taiyang and Yangming stages are both exterior
Which is the half interior/half exterior syndrome?	Shaoyang
What is the hallmark s/sx of a Shaoyang syndrome?	Alternating chills and fever
What is the second stage of a disease progression in the Six Channel Theory?	Yangming *Some schools of thought say Shaoyang is 2nd. I disagree, but I can see the argument for it.*

Diagnostics of Chinese Medicine:
Symptom Analysis and Syndrome Differentiation

How many sub-levels does the Yangming stage have and what are they?	Two. • Jing or channel syndrome • Fu or organ syndrome
How do you tell the Yangming Jing stage from the Fu stage?	Constipation. You only see that in the Fu or Organ version of the Yangming Channel Syndrome.
Why is it a bad thing that a pathogen or evil penetrates to the Yangming stage?	Because Yangming is rich in Qi and Blood and feeds the pathogen really well.
What sets the Shaoyang stage apart from the other stages?	Alternating chills and fever.
What's up with the alternating s/sx in the Shaoyang stage?	Shows you the disease is ½ interior and ½ exterior in its' progression inward.

Sidebar: I've heard experienced practitioners say they feel that ½ and ½ of any s/sx could indicate Shaoyang syndrome. One instructor said she approached bipolar disorder in this way in patients with good results. There is a National Institutes of Health PubMed article supporting this, actually. Check it out here as of this printing: https://www.ncbi.nlm.nih.gov/pubmed/20653162

The Taiyin or Greater Yin syndrome is related to what two channels?	Spleen and Lung
At what stage of the Six Channels do pathogens officially cross into the interior?	Taiyin Stage
At what stage does the body change from a state of excess to a state of deficiency?	At the Taiyin stage. When you shift from exterior to interior you shift from excess to xu.
List the damp cold s/sx in the Taiyin stage.	• Abdominal fullness and/or pain • Nausea and vomiting • No thirst • Pale tongue w/greasy coat • Slow aspect of the pulse

What two organs are under attack when a disease enters the Shaoyin syndrome stage?	Kidney and Heart
What are the two sub-stages of a Shaoyin syndrome?	Shaoyin cold syndrome Shaoyin heat syndrome
Shaoyin cold syndrome looks like what Zangfu diagnosis organ syndrome?	Kidney Yang xu *Look at your Zangfu Combination charts.*
Shaoyin heat syndrome looks much like what Zangfu diagnosis organ syndrome?	Heart/Kidney Disharmony *Look at your Zangfu Combination charts.*
Once a pathogen reaches the Jueyin level in the Six Channel theory, what two organs are under attack?	Liver and Pericardium *Look at your Zangfu Combination charts.*

Write out charts, similar to the ones you did for the Zangfu. Write them over and over again until they get abbreviated into whatever study speak has evolved in your amazing brain.

If you find you don't learn by writing, but by hearing, then do that. Record yourself reading this. Do you. Record it, act it out, dance it, draw it, create an app for it. Whatever kind of learner you are, use the methods that work for you.

But you seriously need to make those charts in some fashion. Great for study, great for clinic (assuming they are some kind of 2D print thing), great for learning. Or create an app. I'd probably buy that.

SECTION 4
Wen Bing or The Four Levels

Wen Bing, or the Four Levels theory, is one of the ways in which you can diagnose and treat diseases in TCM. The Four Levels is designed for identification and treatment of invasions of wind-heat or warm febrile and epidemic diseases (acute externally contracted diseases that are hot in nature).

Onset for these diseases is generally rapid, with fevers and predominant heat signs, diseases are exogenous in nature, are generally associated with specific seasons of the year and can be found grouped in specific locations. The mobile nature of our society, however, can spread a contagious disease further and wider (i.e., H1N1/Swine flu and avian flu epidemics) than was possible when the Warm Disease school of TCM doctors was treating when the theory was first developed during the late Ming and early Qing Dynasty (A.D., 16th C.).

Infection is acquired in warm diseases via respiratory contact, through ingestion of food and in rare cases through skin contact. The respiratory and food-borne routes are by far the most common. Food ingestion will most often lead to a damp heat condition and gastrointestinal problems.

Onset, as previously stated is acute and rapid, but is further broken down into new and hidden onset. New onset warm diseases will often progress through the four stages of the disease. The body's defenses are stimulated by the invasion and a set of reactions (symptoms and signs) appear.

Hidden onset warm disease, however, is the result of previous contact and invasion of the pathogen. Rather than being expelled, the pathogen hides quietly inside the body and waits until conditions are ripe for it to emerge, rather like a terrorist sleeper cell. In these cases, the early stages are skipped and you will see sudden severe symptoms such as high fevers, strong pulse, severe thirst, scanty urine, red tongue, etc. very quickly. One example of this is getting a wind-heat infection in a warmer-than-normal winter, or almost *any* winter in my current town, Austin Texas, then getting a sudden outbreak monster heat signs in the Spring when the warm becomes active with the seasonal rising of Yang qi. (Hint for treatment: don't use exterior formulas because the pathogen is already inside - use clear interior heat formulas instead.)

Regardless of whether the invasion is new or hidden, the exogenous heat associated with warm febrile diseases damages yin and body fluids, so in later stages of Wen Bing deficient heat joins with the excessive heat. Eventually there will be damage to the Zangfu and to their functions.

What follows is by no means a comprehensive look at the Four Levels (Wen Bing), but is a simplified version of the principles of the theory and some treating suggestions. Whole volumes have been written on it and I can't hope to organize it all here. However, you can find more detail about this method of diagnosing and treating by reading *Wen Bing Xue*. Dr. Ye Tian Shi also discussed this theory in his work, *Wen Re Lun* in 1644 A.D.

That said, *should* you learn more about this right now? Maybe not. You'll study a lot about it in classics later in your education.

The Four Levels are:

> Wei or Defensive Qi Level
> Qi Level
> Ying or Nutritive Qi Level
> Xue or Blood Level

CHAPTER 15
Wei Level

The Wei or Defensive level of Qi flows on the outer layers of the body and is yang in relation to the deeper layers. Wei Qi protects the body from pathogens, circulating outside the channels in the skin and muscles. It also warms, moistens and partially nourishes skin and muscle. It adjusts the opening and closing of the pores, regulating sweating and body temperature.

The Lung, with it's ability to disperse and mist, controls Wei Qi. If the Lung Qi is weak, the Wei Qi will probably also be weak. If the Wei Qi is weak, the body's defenses will be weakened. The patient may catch cold easily, and may feel colder more easily than someone with strong Wei Qi.

The Wei stage is usually the initial stage of many infectious and epidemic diseases that are warm in nature. You might think of it as early wind/heat. The initial attack of this type of disease is an attack upon the exterior or surface where the Wei or Defensive Qi guards the body. The skin at the surface and the Wei Qi are closely tied to the Lungs which is why symptoms of wind heat start with Lung related symptoms.

Development of the Wei stage can begin with a mild pathogen and undamaged vital Qi which then pushes the pathogen out of the body. With correct treatment and/or a bit of time, the body will recover. If however the pathogen is severe and/or the vital Qi is weak, improper, non-existent, or delayed treatment can result in the pathogen pushing deeper into the Qi, Ying (Nutritive) and even Xue (Blood) levels. This is a dangerous situation.

Hallmark signs and symptoms are noted by the presence of the pointing finger. ☞

> Fever
> ☞ Chills too, but fever is greater than chills
> ☞ Aversion to cold and possibly wind
> Headache coming from wind/heat attack
> Cough with thick yellow sputum
> Sore throat due to heat in the throat
> Possible sneezing, nasal congestion, sinus drainage
> Very little or no sweating
> Possible slight thirst
> Tongue: Red body with thin white or yellow coat
>> Some sources say red tongue tip and edges (edges here indicate exterior nature)
> Pulse: Floating, rapid

In your classics studies you'll see variations on this theme, but for now, this is plenty. To treat this you could use the herbal formula Yin Qiao San or Sang Ju Yin if you catch this in the early stages. Points you might choose could include Gb 20 (good for all kinds of wind), Li 4, Sj 5, Du 14 (wind and warmth – bleeding and cupping). Sliding cupping would be helpful at Taiyang UB channel. Gua Sha on the Taiyang channel would be good too.

CHAPTER 16
Qi Level

When a pathogen is at the Qi level it has reached the interior of the body, even if it is the most external of the three interior levels. This stage is usually the longest, the broadest, and can have the most severe symptoms, depending on the strength of a person's vital Qi.

If the pathogen is strong and the vital qi is strong, the symptoms can be severe. If the vital Qi is weak, the symptoms may not have such a strong presentation. The Qi level is not considered a life-threatening stage. There is a saying that "*Nobody dies at the Qi level.*"

However, if a pathogen penetrates this far it has reached the interior portion of the body. The warm/heat evil will attach the Zangfu organs and will manifest as internal heat excess. The Upright or Zheng Qi will come under attack as well. This level includes half-in and half-out symptoms such as you find described in the Shaoyang stage of the Six Channel Theory.

Please be aware that pathogens and diseases do not read textbooks or websites and are likely to do unpredictable things! Pathogens might move from Wei to Qi levels, but are just as likely to jump over the Wei stage entirely and get right down to business at the Qi stage.

This is particularly true for hidden pathogens. They tend to manifest quickly at the Qi stage. You might also be treating a person who is in the Ying stage and notice that their symptoms have moved to the Qi stage, which is actually a good thing and shows that the disease is getting more superficial in the body and is on it's way out.

Look for the Four Bigs below. This looks a lot like
the Yangming level in the Six Channel Theory. Symptoms for
the Qi Level will vary depending on which of the organs is
attacked. The most commonly affected are the Lungs, Stomach,
Large Intestine, Gallbladder and Spleen.

Once again, look for the pointing finger to point you to the
hallmark signs/symptoms.

☞ High fever, excessive heat
☞ Profuse sweating
   No chills, no aversion to cold
   Aversion to heat
☞ Big thirst with a desire for cold drinks
   Cough with sticky yellow sputum and maybe chest pain
   Possible asthma due to Lung Qi xu
   Irritability and restlessness with discomfort in all positions
   Concentrated, very yellow urine with strong smell
   Constipation or watery diarrhea
   Stomach discomfort or aching with distention and aversion
   to pressure
   Tongue: Red body, yellow dry coat. Possibly black coat.
☞ Pulse: Rapid, full, could be deep

Notes:
- Lungs attacked:
  If the Lungs are attacked you will probably see a cough with
  yellow phlegm and/or asthma and/or chest pain.

- Heat in the chest:
  You'll see irritability

- Heat in the Stomach:
  You're likely to see profuse sweating, fever, strong thirst for
  cold liquids, and maybe a black tongue coating.

- Heat in the Large Intestines:
  Look for constipation, abdominal pain and "diarrhea,"

which is likely to be intestinal fluids passing through without absorption of nutrients.

There are so many treatment options it's crazy and all of them are dependent on what kind of Qi level attack is going on (heat in the Lungs, heat in the Stomach, dry heat in the Intestines, Gallbladder heat, etc.).

This page intentionally left blank

Diagnostics of Chinese Medicine:
Symptom Analysis and Syndrome Differentiation

CHAPTER 17
Ying Level

When a pathogen reaches the Ying or Nutritive Level it has penetrated to a deeper energetic layer, a depth at which it begins to damage the Yin and affects the Shen. This level normally follows the Wei and Qi levels.

Ying, the nutritive Qi of the body, is viewed as the Qi of Blood and the precursor of blood. It circulates through the blood vessels and Heart. As a result, most of the symptoms affect the Pericardium/Heart and produce interior deficient heat due to the depletion of the Yin.

The key sign to know is highlighted by the finger. Yeah, that's right. I'm giving you the finger. ☞

	S/sx	Notes
	High fever, worse at night	Heat in the interior
	Mental restlessness, irritability, insomnia	Heat is progressing to the Blood level. As blood belongs to the Heart, the Shen is affected producing mental restlessness and insomnia.
	Delirous or illogical speech, plus muddled consciousness	Maybe even coma.
	Thirst/dry mouth, but little desire to drink	Will take small sips to rinse the mouth. This is a symptom of Stomach deficiency.
☞	Red rash or maculopapular lesions on the skin	Small red dots on some parts of the body due to the heat affecting the blood and making it flow recklessly.
	Tongue: Deep red body, yellow coat	Deep red is more heat, yellow coating is also heat. Peeling, thinning, map coat, or

	that could be peeling or no coat	no coat shows Yin xu.
	Pulse: Thin/fine and rapid	Thin and fire show deficiency while rapid shows heat.

Treatment of the Ying stage depends on whether the heat has affected the Pericardium and by how much dryness is showing. Qing Ying Tang is a good formula to start with. Treatment will focus on clearing Ying heat, nourishing Yin, and moving Blood.

CHAPTER 18
Xue Level

Xue is the Chinese word for Blood, so this is also called the Blood Level. The pathogen has entered into the Blood at this stage, the deepest energetic layer. Because the Heart controls the Blood and the Liver stores the Blood, both organs are affected.

Kidneys are also involved now, probably because of the Heart/Fire and Kidney/Water balance relationship. Blood heat is prominent and bleeding signs are evident as a result throughout the body at the skin and organ levels. The blood is disturbed and exhausted. This is a terminal stage of febrile illness and death is usually quick. Symptoms are of both excess heat and deficient yin (because the heat has burned up the yin resources).

And again, diseases don't know they have rules, so a disease may jump over the Ying stage and skip to the blood stage, can be a hidden pathogen and spring up in the Xue stage, etc.

Symptoms include the Ying level s/sx, but some of them are more advanced and severe.

S/sx	Discussion as needed
Fever	
Restlessness, delirium	
Muddled consciousness or coma	
Maculopapular rashes over whole body	All over the body this time – progression from Ying level
Spasms, shaking	Internal Lv wind due to the heat in the final two levels.

☞	Bleeding s/sx and loss of blood. →	•	Vomiting of blood
		•	Nasal bleeding
		•	Blood in stools
		•	Blood in urine
		•	Bleeding under the skin – maculopapular rashes all over the body, in all of the epithelial layers, including the organ epithelial tissues
	Tongue: Deep red/crimson body or purple body	•	Deep red is interior accumulated heat
		•	Purple would indicate more blood stasis
	Pulse: Thin and fast or choppy	•	Thin = deficiency
		•	Fast = heat
		•	Choppy means the blood is moving erratically, the heart is affected.

Note that children progress to Blood heat very rapidly - you might see red bumps or rashes on their faces when they have fevers – but this does not mean they have a febrile disease nor that they have a Blood stage syndrome. You may also see drugs that mimic the rash symptoms. Look for the signs above and for the symptom history to confirm Xue/Blood stage.

As with any of the end stages, whether here or in the Six Channels system of diagnosis, the organs affected can vary greatly as the body shuts down. Treatment depends on what is affected, but as a rule, you can use similar points and formulas for both the Jing and Xue levels. Xi Jiao Di Huang Tang is a good formulary start which nourish Yin and cools Blood. Ou jie - Lotus root - is also is very good for cooling blood. You could use PC 3, 8, 6 (for Shen). Use the Jing Well points to quickly cool the Blood. You're already at emergency stage, so they aren't likely to complain that you are poking the ends of their digits. You could also use SP 10 to help control bleeding out.

A quick thing about Blood heat that isn't likely to be on a test at this stage of your education. Blood heat can come from either excess of deficient causes. If it's an excess cause, it will affect the Heart and Liver. If it is from deficiency, it will affect Liver and Kidney.

Four Levels Theory
Study Questions

Question	Answers
Who developed the Four Levels Theory?	Dr. Ye Tianshi
What aspect of disease is the Four Levels Theory tracking?	Through the layers of the body – defensive layer, Qi layer, nutritive layer, Blood layer
What temperature of pathogenic invasion was Four Levels designed to diagnose and treat?	Warm pathogens that injure the body (which is why they are referred to as "warm injured") – they start with heat s/sx, i.e. wind heat.
What are the characteristics of an epidemic disease that can be classified by the Four Levels theory?	1. Fast onset 2. Fever, likely very high fever, early in the disease 3. Heat signs/symptoms are the primary manifestation 4. Body Fluids and Yin easily damaged due to high fever
What kind of exterior attack does the Wei level resembled?	Exterior wind heat invasion
How would you describe this pathology?	Stagnation of the protective Qi due to the struggle between the protective Qi and Warm-Heat Pathogens, leading to the failure of the lung in dispersing the protective Qi to the surface, nose, throat.
What is the key s/sx of a Wei Qi stage that makes it stand out from the other stages?	Chills and slight aversion to cold

What other s/sx might you see in a Wei Qi stage?	• Fever • Very little or no sweating • Sneezing • Cough • Nasal congestion • Sinus drainage • Sore throat • Headache • Slight increase in thirst • Red tongue tip, might have a thin yellow coating, but could still be white. • Floating, rapid pulse
If you compare the Four Levels to the Six Channels/Stages, which of the Six Stages does a Wei Qi level resemble?	Kinda looks like the Taiyang Zong Feng stage, but there is more heat in the Wei Qi level.
What is the 2nd stage of progression from a Four Levels perspective?	Qi level.
What does the Qi level basically look like if you view it from a Six Channel perspective?	Kind of like the Yangming levels from the Six Channel Theory.
What sets the Qi level apart from the other levels?	The Four Greats or the Four Bigs.
What *are* the Four Greats?	1. Great fever 2. Profuse sweating 3. Big thirst with a preference for cold 4. Great pulse – big, floaty, slippery.
Seriously? Is "floaty" really a pulse word in Chinese medicine?	No, not really. That's just me.

What is the pathology expressed at the Qi level?	Heat from excess and injury to fluids, which is a consequence of the severe struggle between anti-pathogenic Qi and Warm-Heat pathogen.
What is the third level of disease progression in the Four Levels theory?	Ying or nutritive Qi level
What is the pathology of the Ying Level?	Inward progression of protective or Qi level patterns. Blazing heat damages Yin and disturbs the Heart Shen.
What are the four s/sx that indicate the involvement of the Pericardium, Heart and Shen in the Ying Level?	• Insomnia • Irritability • Restlessness • Occasional delirium or muddled consciousness
What is the key s/sx that shows you that the Ying Level is different from the other four levels?	Maculopapular presentations on the skin: Small red dots on *some parts* of the body due to the heat affecting the blood and making it flow recklessly.
How does the maculopapular presentation of the Ying level differ from the maculopapular presentation of the Xue level?	• Ying level: parts of the skin of the body are affected. • Jue level: more broad spread, all over the body, even in the organs.
What is the fourth level of the Four Levels?	• Xue or Blood level
What are the s/sx of a Xue level pathogenic progression?	• Fever • Restlessness • Delirium • Muddled consciousness or

	even coma • Blood loss (internally, due to heat causing reckless bleeding) • Maculopapular lesions all over the body • Deep red or crimson tongue • Thin and fast pulse or choppy pulse.
What organs are involved in the Xue level?	• Heart • Liver • Kidney
What is the pathology of the Xue level?	Warm-heat pathogen penetrates deeply, disturbs and exhausts the blood
Describe the s/sx you could expect to see if you read a differentiation of "Excess Heat in the Blood Level" in a patient's chart	• Fever • Irritation or mania • Purple or dark macular spots on the body • Blood in the stools or urine • Tremors or spasms. Maybe opisthotonos. • Deep red, scarlet, or purplish tongue body • Wiry, fast pulse.
What s/sx could you expect to see if you see "Deficient Heat in the Blood Level" in a patient chart?	• Constant low fever • Five palm heat • Dry mouth and throat • Fatigue • Emaciation • Mild tremors in the extremities • Red or purple tongue with little to no coating • Thin, fast pulse

Diagnostics of Chinese Medicine:
Symptom Analysis and Syndrome Differentiation

SECTION 5
San Jiao Differentiation

The Four Levels detailed the progression of a warm/heat pathogen from external or surface levels to the deep levels of the body. San Jiao Differentiation details the progression of warm/heat pathogens through the upper, middle, and lower jiao.

If you use the two methods together you can get a 3D view of exactly where a pathogen is and where it is heading. It tells you how deep it is from outside to inside and what Jiao it's in. If you also capture a history of how the problem started and how it's changed since the onset, you can also tell what direction it's heading (i.e., getting deeper and more severe going in or coming out of the body and getting better).

This helps you create a good treatment plan, laser targeting your treatments for best accuracy and efficiency. It also helps you understand if the prognosis is getting better or getting worse.

Dr. Wu Ju Tong detailed this method during the Qing Dynasty in his work, *Wen Bing Tiao Bian*.

Some practitioners use these differentiation pattern to diagnose and treat damp plus *heat* pathogens. These are noted below in each of the discussions about the three Jiao patterns and sub patterns. "San" means three in this case and refers to the three jiao. Upper Jiao is above the diaphragm, Middle Jiao is from the diaphragm to the umbilicus, and the Lower Jiao is below the umbilicus.

The Jiaos	Explanation
Upper Jiao	Located above the breathing diaphragm. Includes the organs of the Heart, Lung, and Pericardium
Middle Jiao	Located from the breathing diaphragm to the umbilicus. Includes the organs of the Stomach, Spleen, Large Intestine, and Small Intestine
Lower Jiao	Located from the umbilicus down. Includes the organs of the Liver, Kidney, Bladder, and Uterus

Diagnostics of Chinese Medicine:
Symptom Analysis and Syndrome Differentiation

CHAPTER 19
The Jiao Patterns

This chapter explores the patterns of each of the three Jiao as disease progresses through each in the San Jiao Differentiation diagnostic system.

UPPER JIAO PATTERNS

The upper jiao is located above the breathing diaphragm. Includes the organs of the Heart, Lung, and Pericardium There are three sub-patterns to know about the upper jiao.

Lung Pattern 1 – Pathogens attacking the Lung

This is a disorder of descending and ascending functions of Lung qi due to the influence of an attacking external warm pathogen.

Lu 1 pattern s/sx	Discussion as needed
Fever	
Slight aversion to wind and cold	Looks much like the Wei invasion of the Four Levels. Wind heat type s/sx.
Headache	
Slightly thirsty	
Cough	
Tongue: Thin white coating	
Pulse: Floating, fast	

Lung Pattern 2 – Excessive heat in the Lung

This is a blockage of Lung Qi due to an accumulation of heat in the Lung.

Lung Pattern 2 s/sx	Discussion as needed
Fever	Compare this to the Qi level in the Four Levels.
Sweating	
Thirst	
Dyspnea/trouble breathing	
Tongue: red body, yellow coating	
Pulse: fast	

Upper Jiao damp heat pattern

Upper Jiao damp heat is the early stage of a damp invasion. In this stage damp attacks both the Lungs and the skin. Dampness can also affect the Stomach and Spleen at this stage. At this stage there is less heat/more damp, though heat will predominate if allowed to progress.

Upper Jiao damp heat pattern s/sx	Discussion as needed
Sinus and nasal congestion with yellow discharge, inflammation	Lots of mucus, lots of heat.
Cough with thick yellow mucus	
Swollen lymph glands in neck	
Slight fever or afternoon fevers	
Possible chills and/or sensitivity to cold	
Headache and/or foggy headedness	Heaviness is a big damp s/sx. So is the fogginess.
Sensations of heaviness	
Chest oppression	
Tongue: white coating	
Pulse: Fast	

Diagnostics of Chinese Medicine:
Symptom Analysis and Syndrome Differentiation

Pericardium pattern

This is blockage of the Pericardium by the invasion of heat. As the Pericardium and Heart are so closely related to Shen you will note those signs below.

Pc pattern s/sx	Discussion as needed
Muddled consciousness, mental confusion	Compare this to the Jing/Nutritive Level in the Four Levels.
Delirium	
Retraction of the tongue	
Cold extremities	
Fever	
Tongue: deep red body	
Pulse: thin, rapid	

MIDDLE JIAO PATTERNS

The Middle Jiao is located in the mid-abdomen (breathing diaphragm to umbilicus). The organs of digestion, Stomach, Small Intestine, Large Intestine, and Spleen form the center of the human being, much like Earth is the key element in the classical five elements diagrams. Though the Liver and Gallbladder do reside in this same area they are functionally included in the Lower Jiao.

Fire
Heart
Love

Wood
Liver
Anger

Earth
Spleen
Thought

Metal
Lung
Grief

Water
Kidney
Fear

Sw

There are four Middle Jiao sub-patterns: Stomach pattern, Large Intestine pattern, Spleen pattern, and Middle Jiao damp heat pattern.

Stomach Pattern

This shows as excessive heat in the Stomach.

St pattern s/sx	Discussion as needed
Fever w/o aversion to cold	Many heat s/sx.
Red face and eyes	
Sweating	
Thirst	
Rough or coarse breathing	
Tongue: Dry yellow coat	
Pulse: Large, flooding	

Large Intestine Pattern

Heat accumulation in the Large Intestine.

LI pattern s/sx	Discussion as needed
Fever reaching it's height in the afternoon	Heat symptom
Constipation	Due to dryness in intestine from the heat
Concentrated urine	Could be dark
Tongue: yellow or black coating	Extreme heat
Pulse: deep, strong	Interior and excessive

Spleen Pattern

This is disturbance of the Spleen by damp heat. Compare this to the Middle Jiao Damp Heat Pattern below.

Sp pattern s/sx	Discussion as needed
Fever that persists even after sweating	Cannot disperse due to sticky damp nature of this condition
Distention in the chest and epigastrium	Damp heat keeping Qi from moving in the chest and abdomen
Nausea	Spleen affected by damp
Tongue: thick heavy body and a greasy coating	Thick/heavy body is damp, as is greasy
Pulse: soggy	Soggy is damp

Middle Jiao Damp Heat Pattern

Because the Spleen is so easily weakened by excessive dampness, the Spleen's transformation and transportation functions are damaged by damp heat. The dampness and impairment in the Spleen impacts the Stomach's ability to receive food and water. Muscle tenderness and heaviness is not uncommon because the Spleen cannot keep the muscles and limbs nourished.

Middle Jiao Dampness left untreated can 1) dry and turn into Qi stage of the 4 levels, 2) cool into a cold/damp pattern, or 3) progress to the Lower Jiao.

MJ damp heat pattern s/sx	Discussion as needed
Bloating, gas, indigestion	Typical of Spleen xu/impairment
Loss of appetite	
Nausea, vomiting and diarrhea (possibly with white mucus)	
Jaundice showing in eyes and skin	More so when damp heat is very strong. Face will have a withered dirty dark yellow appearance.
Fever: possibly slight fever, afternoon fever	
Sweating may be reduced	You'd think not, but damp can do this
Heaviness sensations in the limbs	Very common damp symptom
Dry mouth	Heat is burning body fluids, but current damp condition means the body can't process water, so doesn't want more
No desire drink	
Fatigue or lack of energy	Can be Qi xu or damp bogging the body down
Burning sensation upon voiding bladder	Heat and damp passed on to the bladder
Tongue: gray, white and/or yellow coat	Gray could indicate heat and damp – not quite white, not quite black, but headed that way.

Pulse: soft, slow and possibly slippery •	Soft is weakness. Damp can slow the pulse - the pulse is kind of wading through thick mud (damp) here - and can cause the slippery too.

LOWER JIAO PATTERNS

These patterns mostly relate to the Jing and Xue levels from the Four Levels, but Liver fire can be compared to the Qi level also. Lower Jiao pertains to the lower abdomen location in general, but to the function of the Kidney and Liver specifically.

There are three sub-patterns to the Lower Jiao: Kidney, Liver, and Lower Jiao Damp Heat patterns.

Kidney Pattern

The s/sx below occur because of the consumption of Yin by heat. When the Yin is consumed, the result is deficient heat which adds to the problem. You will usually see hypertension due to the consumption of Kidney and Liver Yin which causes the Yang to rise.

Ki pattern s/sx	Discussion as needed
Fever	Looks like Yin deficiency, yes?
Malar flush	
Five palm heat	
Dry mouth and throat	
Fatigue	
Pulse: some kind of deficient pulse type	

Liver Pattern

This is malnutrition of the Liver resulting in inner wind. Remember that Liver and Kidney have the same source, so when one is impaired the other follows. Kidney yin deficiency will generally be evident in this pattern.

Lv pattern s/sx	Discussion as needed
Convulsions and trembling	Inner wind, always related to Liver
Listlessness	Xu s/sx
Palpitations	Shen affected, thus heart affected peripherally.
Tongue: dry, atrophied, deep red body	Severe yin xu
Pulse: weak	Xu

Lower Jiao Damp Heat Pattern

Large Intestines and Bladder are the predominant organs affected so there will be problems with elimination both from the bowels and bladder.

Lower Jiao damp heat pattern s/sx	Discussion as needed
Diarrhea with foul odor and maybe a burning sensation	Damp heat in the Large Intestine
Burning sensation, scant dark-yellow urine	Heat in the Bladder
Yellow smelly vaginal discharge	Heat in the lower jiao
May have genital herpes or PID	PID is pelvic inflammatory disease
Distention in the lower abdomen	Heat and damp retention in the lower jiao
Dizziness	Damp impeding the ascension of clear Qi to the head. Yes, yet another reason for dizziness.
Tongue: Gray white and/or yellow greasy coating	Greasy shows damp, yellow shows heat. Gray could be a transition from yellow to black – heat to even more heat.
Pulse: Soft, rapid, slightly slippery	Soft is deficiency

Study Questions

Question	Answers
What type of pathogenic influence does the San Jiao theory address?	Pathogens that attack with heat – "warm injured" disease.
What type of a disease path does this theory track?	The pathway through the three Jiao, starting at the Upper Jiao.
What organs are the primary attack points in the Upper Jiao?	Lung and Pericardium
Describe the s/sx of an Upper Jiao/Lung Pattern 1 attack.	• Fever • Slight aversion to wind and cold • Headache • Slight thirst • Cough • Thin white tongue coating • Floating, fast pulse
What does the Lung 1 pattern resemble when you compare it to the Four Levels theory?	• Wei level syndrome
The Lung 1 pattern also looks like something you studied in the Eight Principles. What was that?	• Exterior wind/cold syndrome
Describe the s/sx of a Lung 2 Pattern attack in the San Jiao theory of disease.	• Fever • Sweating • Thirst • Dyspnea • Red tongue body with a yellow coat • Fast pulse
What does that look like when you compare it to the Four Levels? (Hint – four bigs)	• Qi level syndrome

What is the definition of the Pericardium sub-pattern	• Blockage of the Pericardium by invasion of heat
What are the s/sx of the Pericardium sub-pattern?	• Muddled consciousness • Delirium • Retraction of the tongue • Cold extremities • Fever • Tongue: deep red • Pulse: thin and rapid
What organs are the primary target in the Middle Jiao patterns?	• Stomach • Large Intestine • Spleen
What is the definition of the Middle Jiao Stomach pattern?	• Excessive heat in the Stomach
What are the s/sx of a Middle Jiao Stomach pattern?	• Fever without aversion to cold • Red face and eyes • Sweating • Thirsty • Rough breathing • Yellow/dry coating on the tongue • Large, flooding pulse
If you compare the Middle Jiao Stomach pattern s/sx to the s/sx you find in the Four Levels, what level does it resemble?	• Qi level – not exactly, but pretty close.
What is the definition of the Middle Jiao Large Intestine pattern?	• Heat accumulation in the Large Intestine

What are the s/sx of the Middle Jiao Large Intestine pattern?	• Fever reaching height in afternoon • Constipation • Concentrated urine • Tongue: yellow to black, dry coating • Deep, strong pulse
What is the definition of the Middle Jiao Spleen pattern?	• Disturbance of Spleen by damp heat
What are the s/sx of the Middle Jiao Spleen pattern?	• Fever which persists even after sweating • Distention in chest and epigastrium • Nausea • Tongue: heavy body, greasy coating • Pulse: soggy
What two patterns do you find the Lower Jiao presentation of the San Jiao Theory?	• Kidney pattern • Liver pattern
What is the definition of the Lower Jiao Kidney pattern?	• Consumption of Yin by heat
What s/sx could you expect to see in the Lower Jiao Kidney pattern?	• Fever • Malar flush • Relatively warm palms/soles • Dry mouth and throat • Fatigue • Pulse: deficient
What is the definition of the Lower Jiao Liver pattern?	• Malnutrition of Liver + inner wind due to Kidney Yin Xu
What s/sx could you expect to see in the Lower Jiao Kidney pattern?	• Convulsions and trembling • Listlessness • Palpitation • Dry, atrophied, and deep red tongue

	• Weak pulse

What is the relationship between the San Jiao and Four Level theories?	• Both explain the progress of a Warm Injured Disease.
	
	   o Four Levels describes progression from superficial to Blood level.
	   o San Jiao describes progression from Upper Jiao down through the Lower

This page intentionally left blank.

Diagnostics of Chinese Medicine:
Symptom Analysis and Syndrome Differentiation

ABOUT THE AUTHOR

Cat Calhoun is a licensed acupuncture practitioner in the State of Texas and soon to be in the State of Florida as well. She attended AOMA Graduate School of Integrative Medicine, earning a Masters degree in Acupuncture and Oriental Medicine. She is passionate about teaching, both formally and informally. Cat has single-handedly created and managed CatsTCMNotes.com since 2008, dispensing notes and clinical pearls to students and practitioners for the past 11 years. She is also passionate about learning, and is currently in love with Master Tung's Acupuncture system.

This book, *Diagnostic Skills in Chinese Medicine: Book 2 – Symptom Analysis and Syndrome Differentiation*, has a companion book for the 1st half of your Diagnostics education in Chinese medicine. Look for it Amazon: *Diagnostic Skills in Chinese Medicine: Book 1 – The Four Diagnostic Skills.* Both of these books are vital for framing your understanding of the diagnostic methods and skills, critical information you need in order to treat effectively in clinic. Both books are available in digital and print format.

Made in the USA
Monee, IL
23 November 2021

82798109R00132